DE

ESSENTIALS
OF
HOSPITAL
RISK
MANAGEMENT

Edited by

Barbara J. Youngberg, J.D., R.N.
Director of Insurance and Risk Management
University Hospital Consortium, Inc.
Oakbrook Terrace, Illinois

AN ASPEN PUBLICATION®
Aspen Publishers, Inc.
Rockville, Maryland
1990

Library of Congress Cataloging-in-Publication Data

Essentials of hospital risk management/edited by Barbara J. Youngberg.
p. cm.
Includes bibliographies and index.
ISBN: 0-8342-0098-8
1. Hospitals--Risk management. 2. Tort liability of hospitals.
3. Insurance, Physicians' liability. I. Youngberg, Barbara J.
[DNLM: 1. Financial Management.
2. Hospital Administration--United States. WX 157 E78]
RA971.38.E88   1989   362.1'1'0681--dc20   DNLM/DLC
for Library of Congress
89-17586
CIP

Editorial Services: Marsha Davies

Library of Congress Catalog Card Number: 89-17586
ISBN: 0-8342-0098-8

Printed in the United States of America

1 2 3 4 5

This book was made possible through the support and encouragement of the University Hospital Consortium, Inc., an alliance of academic medical centers throughout the country. It is dedicated to all the members of the Consortium and to all of their staff, who strive to achieve excellence in health care through quality of service.

Table of Contents

Contributors

James D. Blinn
Actuary
Tillinghast, Nelson & Warren
Skokie, Illinois

Josephine Goode-Johnson
Executive Director
University of Maryland Medical
  Service System
Baltimore, Maryland

Catherine T. Hartlieb
Senior Vice President—
  Production/Marketing
Alexander & Alexander, Inc.
Chicago, Illinois

Sandra L. Jesser, RN, MA
Risk Manager
UCLA Medical Center
Los Angeles, California

Tom M. Jones, Esq.
Partner
McDemott, Will & Emery
Chicago, Illinois

Rodney Klein
Vice President—Finance
University Hospital Consortium
Oakbrook Terrace, Illinois

Deborah Korleski
Risk Manager
Thomas Jefferson University
  Hospital
Philadelphia, Pennsylvania

A. Michele Kuhn
Director, Risk Management
Presbyterian-University Hospital
  of Pittsburgh
Pittsburgh, Pennsylvania

Elizabeth A. Lee, RN, MSPH
Hospital Risk Manager for Loss
  Prevention
The North Carolina Memorial
  Hospital
Chapel Hill, North Carolina

Pamela Ann Lockowitz, MS, RN
Regional Claims Manager
Multi-Systems Agency, Ltd.
Bannockburn, Illinois

Ann R. Mansfield, RN, MS
Director, Risk Management
University of Wisconsin
  Hospital and Clinics
Madison, Wisconsin

Charles M. O'Brien
Administrator
Georgetown University Hospital
Washington, DC

M. Ross Oglesbee, Esq.
Hospital Attorney
The North Carolina Memorial
Hospital
Chapel Hill, North Carolina

Grena Porto-Spillmann
Risk Manager
University Hospital
Stony Brook, New York

Ann L. Schoofs, RRA
Graduate Student in Health
Systems Engineering
University of Wisconsin
Madison, Wisconsin

Michael D. Sheppard
Risk Manager
Metropolitan Rail
Chicago, Illinois

Cecelia E. Yeaton
Assistant Administrator of Risk
Management
University Hospital of Brooklyn
Brooklyn, New York

**Barbara J. Youngberg, J.D.,
BSN, MSW**
Director of Insurance and Risk
Management
University Hospital Consortium
Oakbrook Terrace, Illinois

M. Michael Zuckerman, Esq.
Director of Risk Management
and Insurance
Thomas Jefferson University
Philadelphia, Pennsylvania

Foreword

Health care risk management is an important subject these days as hospitals and other health care institutions confront the increasingly complex legal environment of the 1980s and 1990s. In reality, however, risk management is but one method of navigating around the iceberg of accountability that health care institutions confront in their dealing with the public.

In the future, wc can expect that government agencies, consumers, and professional liability insurers will increasingly be asking what each institution is doing with regard to providing an environment that is as safe as is humanly possible from both system errors and human errors. Risk management is an organized response that focuses attention on issues of quality and encourages the development of management and systems expertise for identifying, within the institution, systems and human errors that can and should be corrected. While the public's dream of a single index of quality within an institution may be quite far off, an effective risk management program can and should be one major element in the hospital's overall quality control program, providing quality management for its medical and professional staff, ensuring quality control over the hospital's board, and promising quality control for the management of the institution.

Essentials of Hospital Risk Management, I believe, will provide an overview of how effective risk programs are established within institutions. And while risk management is often a local issue, and no institution can be expected to follow any cookbook approach, I believe that this book can provide guideposts for the establishment of a comprehensive quality program within any institution.

This book is an outgrowth of an activity undertaken by the University Hospital Consortium (an alliance of academic medical centers nationwide) in an attempt to develop for its members professional liability and risk management programs and standards on a national level. The need to have some uniformity in outcomes for risk management programs among many diverse institutions has led us to put together this book. We believe it can be of use to all health care providers, offering them guidelines and tools for establishing, organizing, and controlling all aspects of risk within their institutions. We are pleased to share this effort with you.

Charles M. O'Brien
Administrator
Georgetown University Hospital

Preface

Today's professional hospital risk manager faces new and exciting challenges. Though the risk manager's job traditionally centered around preserving the financial integrity of the institution and making its environment safe, the job's focus has now broadened to include the prevention of patient injury and the promotion of quality service. The competitive environment of today's health care industry, coupled with rising malpractice verdicts, defense costs, and insurance premiums, has forced hospital administrators and physicians to respond by placing increased emphasis on developing systems to monitor, promote, and guarantee quality of service.

Licensing agencies and professional organizations now describe minimum standards for risk management programs. These standards include active medical staff involvement and support, support of the administrative or governing body, appropriate operational linkages between the departments of quality assurance and risk management, and an increased focus on the evaluation of high-risk activity occurring within the health care setting.

Though the directives are clear, their implementation can be difficult. The purpose of this book is to provide guidelines and tools that will assist the risk manager or health care executive to analyze his or her current programs and develop new programs that will be more sensitive to quality of care issues. It is my belief that once the focus shifts from finances to quality, with the prevention of patient harm or injury being the focus, hospital staff and physicians will engage more in the risk management process (and in many instances will feel less threatened by it).

Many of the contributors to this book are actively involved in hospital risk management and have shared tools developed within their institutions to more fully evaluate and monitor the quality of care rendered. Some of these programs took years to develop. We are optimistic that their inclusion will assist readers in shortening this development process within their institutions. Other contributors have years of experience in the areas of hospital law, hospital professional liability insurance, health care actuarial science, and risk financing. I felt that their technical expertise would make a critical contribution to this book by assisting professional risk managers to function in their new and demanding roles.

chapter 1

The Emergence of a Profession

Deborah Korleski

In order to understand the development of risk management as a distinct profession within the health care industry, it is necessary to examine how and why it has emerged. In large part, health care risk management emerged in response to the malpractice crisis of the mid-1970s. This crisis prompted action on various fronts to ensure the continued availability of malpractice insurance for hospitals and physicians. The initial emphasis of risk management in the hospital setting focused on risk financing and safety/environmental risk control techniques. Today, the discipline of health care risk management encompasses not only these areas but also a multitude of exposures related to the provision of patient care. This chapter traces the development of health care risk management from its emergence in the 1970s to the profession it has become today.

MALPRACTICE CRISIS

Medical malpractice received a great deal of attention in the early 1970s when a crisis emerged due to the lack of availability of liability insurance. Most insurance carriers increased premiums at alarming rates, and others stopped writing malpractice coverage altogether, thereby shrinking market capacity. The increased frequency and severity of malpractice claims were the primary factors precipitating these actions. Insurers found themselves unable to adequately predict the frequency of claims or to adequately price this line of insurance.

A number of studies were undertaken to determine the extent of the crisis and to identify solutions. One of the first studies conducted was at the direction of President Richard Nixon in 1971. The Department of Health, Education, and Welfare Secretary's Commission on Medical Malpractice set out to identify and evaluate the causes of malpractice claims, the effectiveness of the professional liability insurance system, the effectiveness of current legal mechanisms for compensating injured parties, and the attitudes of the general public.

The Secretary's Commission found that malpractice claims were primarily the result of injuries or adverse results of medical treatment. The commission did, however, acknowledge that not all injuries were due to negligence, and not all injuries were preventable. These findings were based on the results of studies concerning the incidence of iatrogenic injuries. One study revealed that 7.5 percent of reviewed medical records showed evidence of iatrogenic injury. Based on these studies, there were many more injuries than claims. A significant commission finding was that the severity of the injury was more apt to be the determinative factor in deciding whether a claim would arise. The commission concluded that the most effective way to reduce the frequency and severity of injuries was to develop medical injury prevention programs in every health care institution.[1]

Similar conclusions were drawn by the 1977 American Bar Association Commission on Medical Professional Liability, which stated that "a reduction in the frequency and severity of avoidable incidents which result in injuries to patients is of great importance." Based on its inquiries, it concluded that with few exceptions, the primary focus of patient safety programs in hospitals was improving the physical environment and was not aimed at medically caused injuries. It recommended that the hospital industry and the medical profession work together to develop ways to prevent avoidable medically related injuries to patients.[2]

A report from the Committee on Law and Medicine of the Bar Association of the City of New York also commented on the need to prevent injuries and presented the recommendation that hospitals establish medical injury prevention programs aimed at investigating the causes of injuries and developing measures to minimize the risks.[3]

In an effort to ease the malpractice crisis, state legislators enacted a variety of laws designed to establish limits on the amount of awards, set up arbitration screening panels, revise the contingency fee systems, and modify the collateral source rules. These mechanisms seemingly provided a short-term solution to the crisis, but within less than a decade, many of these reforms were challenged on constitutional grounds or in some cases (e.g., the use of arbitration panels) had only made the system more cumbersome. From an insurance perspective, various alternative risk financing mechanisms were created, namely, joint underwriting associations, state-administered compensation funds, and other insurance pooling devices.[4] By and large, these risk financing mechanisms have endured, and many of them are still available today.

The underlying causes of the increase in malpractice claims, however, were not addressed by these reforms. These underlying causes include technological advances in medicine, which carry increased risk of injury; the deterioration of the physician-patient relationship; patients' unrealistic expectations as to treatment outcomes; and the increased likelihood of errors due to the increased numbers of individuals involved in patient care.[5] The increased focus on health care, due to individual hospitals' marketing strategies of emphasizing the "we can do anything better" philosophy, has also increased the public's expectations related to health care.

This climate of increasing liability claims and decreasing availability of liability insurance, coupled with increasing pressure to contain health care costs, propelled hospitals into action. These actions included implementing alternative risk financing techniques (i.e., self-insurance) and developing more comprehensive risk management programs.

Reaction to the malpractice crisis of the 1970s ensured the continued availability of liability insurance; however, insurers continued to experience malpractice losses that exceeded premiums. Favorable investment income tempered the effects of these losses until interest rates declined, necessitating substantial increases in premiums or changes in the types of coverage available. This eventually led to another malpractice crisis in the mid-1980s as the frequency and severity of claims continued to increase and the costs of liability insurance correspondingly escalated.[6] This crisis also saw a change in individual hospitals' assumption of risk, with individual institutional financing often well in excess of a million dollars. The emergence of this second crisis provided additional support for health care risk management and helped hospitals to recognize the need for internal program development.

RISK MANAGEMENT PROGRAM DEVELOPMENT

The term "risk management," although familiar to insurance professionals and to industry, was not easily understood or readily accepted in the health care industry. For some hospitals, risk management programs were initiated to comply with an insurance carrier's requirement, as a condition of coverage. Often these programs lacked the necessary commitment of the hospital's administration, governing board, and medical and other professional staff to truly be effective. Compounding this was the delegation of the risk management function to persons without prior risk management knowledge or experience. Guidance from the American Hospital Association (AHA) helped to foster the acceptance of risk management in health care. The AHA defined risk management as the "science for the identification, evaluation, and treatment of the risk of financial loss" and encouraged hospitals to implement risk management programs as a key solution to malpractice problems.[7]

Through a series of workshops conducted in 1977, the AHA identified the basic elements of risk management programs in existence at that time. It also described areas that required expansion and improvement. The AHA staff found that the risk manager was someone whose training or background was in hospital administration, insurance, or safety engineering. Prior to assuming responsibility for risk management, many were already employed by the hospital in finance, personnel, research, education, nursing, security, or claims management positions. Risk managers reported to the chief executive officer or an associate administrator and only devoted about 50 percent of their time to risk management activities, which included the identification, evaluation, and treatment of the risk of financial loss; the receipt and investigation of incident reports; analysis and evaluation of exposure trends; recommendations and monitoring of specific treatment in incidents of injury; and education. Many risk managers also participated in claims management, insurance evaluation, and purchasing.

Risk managers identified as imperative to an effective hospital-wide liability control system the following: training of all medical, executive, volunteer, and employee staffs in the processes of liability control; reducing incidents of patient injury; and identifying potentially injurious events and correcting them. The lack of cooperation of the medical staff, the lack of authority necessary for effective analysis and follow-up, and the lack of awareness and understanding of a risk control system were cited as barriers to successful implementation of an effective program.[8]

Initial risk management efforts in hospitals focused on the physical environment of the hospital, equipment safety, and staff training.[9] This "safety model" emphasized injury prevention but was limited in scope and did not deal effectively with injuries resulting from physician activities. Recognizing that most claims result from "people failures" (and that the most costly claims arise from patient injury during the course of rendering care), a systems approach evolved, emphasizing coordination and cooperation between the hospital and the physician staff.[10] Of utmost concern was the professional liability exposure, as hospitals faced increasing liability for the actions of its employees and physicians. The "patient injury" model emphasized the importance of improving the quality of patient care as an integral component of risk management and mandated the active participation of the medical staff in risk management activities.[11] The adoption of this approach to risk management has evolved gradually.

As the second malpractice crisis emerged in the early 1980s, there was renewed interest in risk management. In 1980 the American Society for Healthcare Risk Management (ASHRM) of the AHA was formed in response to the need for a professional association for the growing number of hospital risk managers. At that time, the AHA estimated that 51.5 percent of the nation's hospitals had organized risk management programs.[12]

In 1985 the General Accounting Office of the federal government initiated a study of medical malpractice claims and recommended that risk management programs be expanded and strengthened.[13] As of 1987, six states had passed legislation requiring hospitals to establish internal risk management programs. These statutes were designed to minimize patient injury by ensuring the competency of health care providers and establishing systems to identify and correct problems that have the potential to harm patients.[14] Further recognition of the importance of risk management was evidenced by the development of risk management standards by the Joint Commission on Accreditation of Healthcare Organizations. These standards require implementation of risk reduction functions that include the active involvement of the medical staff.[15] ASHRM, along with state and local risk management associations, contributed to the development of health care risk management and helped to shape its direction. In 1987 ASHRM drafted language for a model risk management program.[16] Since its emergence in the mid-1970s, health care risk management has grown in importance, and its scope of activities has expanded to address all areas of potential liability exposure to the institution.

RISK MANAGEMENT PROGRAM DESCRIPTION (THE IDEAL)

Although the actual implementation of a risk management program is dependent upon the unique characteristics of the individual hospital, there are essential components necessary for an effective program. These components include

- Senior administration and governing body commitment and support, evidenced through the appropriation of sufficient resources to manage risk management activities
- Designation of a risk manager (and risk management staff as appropriate) to coordinate all aspects of the program and to communicate loss prevention activities to key administrative personnel, who
  —is part of the administrative team and has direct access or reports directly to the chief executive officer or chief operating officer

—has access to all hospital and medical staff data

—is knowledgeable about hospital operations (including clinical practice, if possible), insurance and legal issues, and possesses good communication skills

- Support of the medical staff and their participation in reporting adverse outcomes, incidents, or any event that may result in a claim (which information should be incorporated into the physician reappointment process)
- Integration with quality assurance and sharing of information and findings in the monitoring and evaluation of the quality of patient care
- Establishment of reporting mechanisms to identify unusual incidents, unexpected outcomes, or potential risks, utilizing not only incident reports but also occurrence or generic screening, attorney requests for medical records, patient complaints, billing office complaints, and so on
- Early investigation of all serious unanticipated or unexpected outcomes resulting in patient injury
- Prospective and retrospective analyses of risk exposures for trends or patterns
- Implementation of prevention programs to minimize patient injuries or loss
- Education of physician, nursing, and hospital staff to promote awareness of risk management and liability control
- Review of new ventures, programs, services, and technology to address any risk management implications associated with these activities
- Meetings with established medical staff and hospital committees for the receipt and review of risk management information
- Risk financing
- Claims management

An effective risk management program covers all aspects of hospital operations. To effectively implement the program requires the cooperation of administration, medical staff, nursing, and department heads. The goal is to be proactive, identifying problems before an injury or loss occurs and taking action to prevent or minimize its effects. To achieve this goal means establishing early warning systems, targeting clinical areas or practices that present the greatest exposure to liability, and implementing preventive action to minimize the risk associated with these activities. Risk management is a valuable resource whose purpose is to preserve the assets of the institution while contributing to the hospital's mission of providing quality care to patients.

CONCLUSION

In the mid-1970s a crisis emerged in the availability of liability insurance for health care providers. In response to this crisis came the development of risk management programs in the health care environment. In the mid-1980s a new insurance crisis emerged in the affordability of liability insurance, prompting even more health care institutions to seek alternative risk financing mechanisms and to strengthen their risk management programs. The underlying factors contributing to these crises are still present today, only to a much greater degree. Today's risk manager faces a more litigious health care consumer, who often equates a bad outcome with malpractice; continuing technological advances, with their inherent risks; and a continual emergence of new areas of liability as new services are developed (e.g., home care, health maintenance organizations) and court decisions rendered. Risk management has evolved to meet these challenges and has developed into a unique and comprehensive profession that will continue to advance in the coming decade.

The essence of risk management was captured by William Ryan in an article entitled "An Aspect of the Growth and Development of Hospital Risk Management":

> In assessing his or her role and its value to the health care facility, the risk manager should keep three things in mind: (1) that risk management is a comprehensive teamwork activity and that he or she is a participant in an institution-wide process involving every department, employee, and medical staff member, (2) that his or her role encompasses the recognition of, prevention or containment of, and recovery from loss, and (3) that he or she is a leader in molding attitudes throughout the institution toward the risk management process.[17]

NOTES

1. Department of Health, Education, and Welfare, *Report of the Secretary's Commission on Medical Malpractice,* DHEW Publication No. (OS) 73-88 (Washington, D.C.: Government Printing Office, 1973), pp. 25, 51, 61.
2. American Bar Association, *1977 Report of the Commission on Medical Professional Liability* (Chicago: American Bar Association, 1977), pp. 25, 27, 30.
3. Bar Association of the City of New York, *Report on the Medical Malpractice Insurance Crisis* (New York: The Committee on Law and Medicine, 1975), p. 91.
4. "Rx for the Medical Malpractice Crisis," *Journal of American Insurance* (Summer 1976): 23–30.
5. D. Mechanic, "Some Social Aspects of the Medical Malpractice Dilemma," in *The Duke Law Journal Symposium on Medical Malpractice* (Cambridge, Mass.: Ballinger Publishing Co., 1977), p. 3.

6. American Medical Association, *Special Task Force on Professional Liability and Insurance* (Chicago: American Medical Association, 1984).

7. T. Dankmyer and J. Groves, "Taking Steps for Safety's Sake," *Hospitals* 51 (May 16, 1977): 60; S. Holloway and A. Sax, "The AHA Urges, Aids Hospitals to Adopt Effective Risk Management Plans," *Hospitals* 51 (May 16, 1977): 57.

8. Y. Bryant and A. Korsak, "Who Is the Risk Manager and What Does He Do?" *Hospitals* 52 (January 16, 1978): 42–43.

9. T. Chittenden, "Role of Physician in Malpractice Needs More Careful Exploration," *Hospitals* 51 (May 16, 1977): 53.

10. Maryland Hospital Education Institute, *Controlling Hospital Liability: A Systems Approach* (Chicago: American Medical Association, 1976), p. 2; American College of Surgeons, *Patient Safety Manual: A Guide for Establishing a Patient Safety System in Your Hospital* (Chicago: American College of Surgeons, 1979), p. 4.

11. J. Orlikoff and A. Vanagunas, *Malpractice Prevention and Liability Control for Hospitals* (Chicago: American Hospital Association, 1988), pp. 34–35.

12. D. Roberts, J. Shane, and M. Roberts, *Confronting the Malpractice Crisis: Guidelines for the Obstetrician-Gynecologist* (Kansas City: Eagle Press, 1983), p. 21.

13. U.S. General Accounting Office, *Medical Malpractice: A Framework for Action*, GAO/HRD-87-73 (Washington, D.C.: General Accounting Office, 1987), pp. 16–17.

14. S. Salpeter, "State Statutes Take Aim at Malpractice Insurance Crisis," *Perspectives in Healthcare Risk Management* (Summer 1987): 12–13.

15. Joint Commission on Accreditation of Healthcare Organizations, *Accreditation Manual for Hospitals* (Chicago: Joint Commission on Accreditation of Healthcare Organizations, 1988), p. 121.

16. American Society for Healthcare Risk Management, "Model Language for a Healthcare Risk Management Program," *Perspectives in Healthcare Risk Management* (Spring 1987): 23–24.

17. W. Ryan, "An Aspect of the Growth and Development of Hospital Risk Management," *Perspectives in Hospital Risk Management* 3, no. 1 (Spring 1983): 11.

PART I

Setting Up a Strong Department

The *risk management process* requires the participation of all hospital and medical staff members to succeed. Establishing a risk management department to coordinate this process centralizes, formalizes, and expands ongoing loss control activities in a hospital. The concept of risk management must be "sold" to the board, the administration, and the medical staff for the program to succeed. Once the concept is sold, care must be taken so that the department is developed to meet the needs of the institution.

The size and organization of the risk management department are influenced by many factors, including the method of risk financing, size of the institution, complexity of the risk, regulatory requirements of the state, and scope of the risk manager's responsibility. Although some general guidelines are presented in Chapter 2, there is no single correct configuration of a risk management department.

Establishing a risk management department will require the institution to invest money and time. Some of the costs will be nonrecurring. However, the benefits of the program, if successful, will greatly outweigh the costs.

Analyzing the Needs of the Institution and Establishing a Risk Management Department

Grena Porto-Spillmann

The goals of risk management in the health care setting are to prevent patient injury and prevent or limit financial loss to the institution. These goals are accomplished by identifying areas of risk, analyzing and evaluating risks, and treating and managing those risks.

Prior to the liability crisis of the early 1970s, programs to prevent patient injury existed in hospitals in an informal and decentralized way. For example, nursing departments practiced techniques to prevent patient falls, biomedical engineering departments conducted inspections of patient care equipment to prevent patient injury, and medical staff conducted morbidity and mortality reviews to identify complications and deaths that could have been prevented. However, these activities were carried out randomly, not as part of a hospital program to prevent patient injury and minimize financial loss.

After the liability crisis of the 1970s, hospitals began to incorporate departmental efforts to prevent patient injury into hospital-wide initiatives, which were then called risk management programs. Thus, risk management programs were born of existing practices that were expanded, formalized, and centralized. Hospitals began to apply techniques that had been practiced for many years by the business world to address the problems of loss prevention and management.

The development of risk management systems and formalized risk management departments in hospitals has also been influenced by regulatory factors. The federal government has taken a strong interest in reducing the cost of health care and presumably in monitoring and guaranteeing

11

quality. In addition to enacting changes in reimbursement systems, the federal and state governments have taken steps to reduce costs by mandating various risk management practices in health care. The Health Care Quality Improvement Act of 1986 addressed the issue of credentialing. The Joint Commission on Accreditation of Healthcare Organizations (Joint Commission) has for the first time promulgated standards of risk management, which became effective in January 1989. Several states have enacted additional regulatory requirements in risk management and related areas such as quality assurance and physician credentialing. Thus, there are now many compelling reasons for establishing a strong, hospital-wide risk management department.

By establishing a risk management department, a hospital formalizes, centralizes, and expands existing loss prevention initiatives. It is important to realize that while the formation of a risk management department provides focus for these efforts, the success of the programs will depend on the degree to which all hospital departments and staff understand and participate in the process. Although the risk management department may prescribe the methods by which the goals of the program are attained, the actual techniques of risk management will continue to be practiced by the caregiver and hospital staff. Therefore, it is important to establish a risk management program that integrates all loss prevention activities in the hospital and enlists the participation of all hospital departments and staff. The purpose of this chapter is to provide the administrator or risk manager charged with establishing a risk management department (or with evaluating a currently existing program) with a step-by-step formula to achieve this. The chapter covers the process from gaining administrative support for the program to hiring the right people to staff the department.

GAINING ADMINISTRATIVE SUPPORT FOR THE RISK MANAGEMENT PROGRAM

For any new hospital program to succeed, it must have the proper support from the participants. This often involves overcoming misconceptions individuals have about what the program is. Thus, the first step in setting up a risk management program involves conducting an educational campaign to inform the hospital community about it. Administrators and board members often view risk management with suspicion and believe that it merely duplicates existing programs such as quality assurance. Cost considerations related to establishing a program are also considered. Of course, administrators and board members who have been exposed to the liability crisis in recent years understand that there is indeed a very real need to limit patient injuries and the costs associated with them. However, administrators and board members may be uncertain about how risk management will accomplish this.

The hospital administrator or risk manager should be prepared to educate board members about the risk management process and how it resembles and differs from quality assurance. Board members should be taught that both risk management and quality assurance have a common ground, particularly in the area of risk identification and prevention. However, each process treats risk differently and has different objectives. Quality assurance tends to be concerned with trends or patterns that are suggestive of substandard care. Risk management, though, would focus on risks as potential liability exposures and would evaluate each one for its impact on the institution's financial position, regardless of whether a trend or pattern exists. The primary goal of quality assurance is to improve care, while risk management is concerned not only with improving patient care and preventing harm to patients but also with limiting the institution's financial liability exposure. This is accomplished by early management and resolution of actual or potential claims and by the recognition and control of negligent practices of staff that have or can lead to lawsuits.

One way to clarify the relationship between risk management and quality assurance is to provide an example of how the two processes might interact. Assume that risk management and quality assurance share a system of risk identification that involves generic outcome screening. One of the screens is a baby born with low Apgar scores. Both risk management and quality assurance consider this a risk requiring further investigation. Quality as surance would evaluate this risk for evidence of substandard care. This would probably be done through the peer review process. If no evidence of substandard care was identified and no pattern or trend found, quality assurance would take no further action. This event would be considered an isolated occurrence, and the decision might be made to simply watch for further occurrences of this type.

Risk management, however, would consider this a serious potential liability exposure for the hospital, even if no trend or pattern existed. In addition to evaluating this risk for evidence of substandard care, the risk manager would probably conduct an extensive investigation of the facts of the case in preparation of anticipated litigation, including an evaluation of actual or potential injury. This investigation is not a peer review function. Even if the care was found to be adequate by a peer review system, the risk manager might still consider this a liability exposure, especially if the baby sustained injury, and might conduct an investigation. A claim file would be established, and this exposure would be included in various calculations which would impact on professional liability claims tracking and on the institution's financial position. This event would continue to be treated as a risk until no threat of liability exposure existed.

If the care was found to be substandard, both risk management and quality assurance would take action. This might take the form of cooperative efforts to change policy and procedure and the implementation of other corrective actions. Furthermore, the risk manager might begin an investigation of all of the facts related to this incident, in anticipation of potential litigation.

The board and administrators should also be taught that in addition to preventing, controlling, and financing risks associated with patient care, risk management has other areas of responsibility as well. Risk managers may also be responsible for workers' compensation programs, all aspects of insurance management, propery loss control programs, contract review, and monitoring of all medical-legal problems.

Board members and administrators should be made to understand that risk management does not replace quality assurance. There are a number of quality assurance issues that are identified and resolved through the quality assurance process that have no impact on potential liability for the institution and with which risk management would not be concerned. Quality assurance seeks to improve quality of care to the best level possible, while risk management is primarily concerned with achieving the legal standard of care. Risk management and quality assurance are complementary processes. They overlap in their goals of improving patient care and preventing patient injury, but also differ in their methods and in other goals and objectives. Figure 2-1 depicts the functions of risk management and quality assurance and their relationship to each other.

Once board members and administrators understand the risk management process and its relationship to quality assurance, the argument for cost-effectiveness can be made. The board and administration should understand that one of the goals of risk management is to prevent or limit the financial liability of the institution. An effective risk management program will reduce financial loss and thereby, if successful, will pay for itself.

The institution's claims history, premium history, and the costs of the use of consultants for these services can all be used as compelling arguments in favor of establishing an in-house risk management department.

Finally, the need for regulatory compliance can be used as an argument for establishing a risk management department. Although regulatory requirements usually compel hospitals to establish a risk management process rather than a department, establishing a department is the most cost-effective way of satisfying the requirement.

Once the decision to establish a department has been made, it will be important to gain administrative support for the risk management program. One way to accomplish this is to involve key administrators in the early

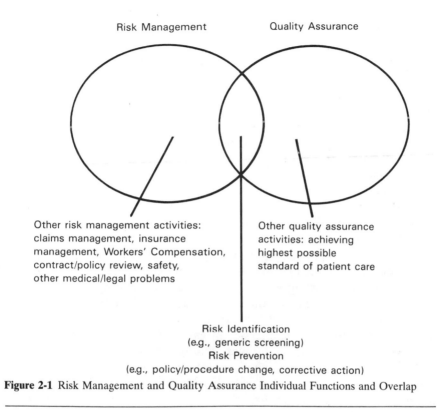

Figure 2-1 Risk Management and Quality Assurance Individual Functions and Overlap

planning of the program and in the search for a qualified risk manager. Among the individuals who should be involved are the medical director, the physician director of quality assurance, the director of nursing, and the chief financial officer.

GAINING SUPPORT FROM THE MEDICAL STAFF

Physicians are often suspicious of the risk management process and may not initially support the program. Often they feel that risk management is really just another way to blame physicians for patient care problems. Sometimes they believe that the role of the risk manager is to make the physicians assume as much of the financial burden of a liability claim as possible. The fact that physicians and hospitals are often insured by different carriers and represented by different attorneys may contribute to the animosity many physicians feel toward hospital risk management programs.

A well-organized educational campaign combined with a commitment by the hospital to build a cooperative relationship with its medical staff can overcome any resistance physicians may feel toward risk management. First, however, the hospital must resolve that it will not use the risk management program as a way of exploiting medical staff in liability claims for the benefit of the hospital. This is often not an easy resolution to make or to keep due to pressure from insurance carriers and defense attorneys. However, the hospital has far more to lose by jeopardizing the cooperation and commitment of its medical staff in regard to risk management, quality assurance, and other essential quality monitoring functions.

The administrator can begin by educating the medical staff about the risk management process and its goals. The help of the medical director and the physician director of quality assurance can be a valuable tool in this effort. As with the board of directors and administration, there may be questions about how quality assurance differs from risk management. These can be handled in the same manner described in the previous section.

There are two important points to emphasize when gaining support from physicians. The first is that the risk management program offers a multi-faceted service consisting of advice on a number of topics, including informed consent, documentation, patients' rights, preventing patient injuries, refusal and withdrawal of treatment, confidentiality, communications from attorneys, malpractice litigation, "Do Not Resuscitate" orders, and other medical-legal topics. The second point is that supporting and participating in the risk management program will not require a large outlay of physicians' time. Unlike quality assurance, risk management does not require physicians to perform extensive chart audits on a regular basis. This is an important consideration, particularly for physicians with private practices outside the hospital.

OTHER CONSIDERATIONS IN GAINING SUPPORT FOR A RISK MANAGEMENT PROGRAM

There may also be some resistance to the implementation of a risk management program on the part of other staff members. For example, nurses and other licensed professionals often fear that involvement in a liability claim will jeopardize their licenses. Therefore, they may be reluctant to report liability problems or to support risk management efforts. Again, the best approach to dealing with this problem is education about what risk management is and how it works. It should be emphasized that risk management is a service provided by the hospital to protect the hospital and its employees from liability.

Finally, the administrator or risk manager should be aware that some resistance to implementation of a risk management program may come from staff members who perceive this as an intrusion into their areas of expertise or authority. This is sometimes the case with quality assurance staff in hospitals in which the risk manager's role is limited to risk identification and prevention. The best way to deal with this problem is to clearly delineate from the start of the program who will be responsible for what functions, and how these areas will be expected to interact with the risk management function. This is discussed in greater depth later in this chapter and in subsequent chapters in this book.

ANALYZING THE HOSPITAL'S NEEDS

Once the decision has been made to establish a risk management program, and the support of the administration and hospital and medical staff has been enlisted, it is necessary to determine what the hospital's risk management needs are. A number of factors should be considered, including:

What Type of Risk Financing Arrangements Does the Institution Have?

A self-insured institution will have to invest in the proper staff to administer and maintain the self-insurance program. Such a hospital is in many ways functioning as its own insurance carrier and must make arrangements to provide its own claims and risk management services. Many of these services can be provided by outside consultants; however, the hospital will also require a full-time risk manager with one or more support people to coordinate the program. In addition, the risk manager must carefully monitor the use of consultants to make certain the arrangement remains cost-effective. Also, the risk manager must provide direction to consultants to ensure that the necessary services are received. If the hospital intends to limit the use of consultants, additional staff in the risk management department will be required.

A commercially insured hospital can expect to receive much of its claims management and some of its risk management services from the carrier. Such a hospital may not need to maintain a large risk management staff. However, commercially insured hospitals still must have organized risk management programs. Many professional liability and excess carriers require such a program as a condition of coverage. Also, the availability of such coverage varies from year to year, and no assumption should be made that a carrier providing coverage and risk and claims management services will be willing to continue to do so in the future. Therefore, commercially insured hospitals still need to have an organized risk management program, although the size of the staff will be smaller than for the self-insured hospital.

What Is the Size of the Institution?

Large hospitals (400 beds or more) will almost certainly require a full-time risk manager with one or more support people. Such institutions tend to offer more complex services and often are partially or fully self-insured.

Small hospitals (200 beds or less) often do not require full-time risk managers. These institutions may hire a part-time risk manager or assign the responsibility for a risk management program to an administrator or staff member with other assigned duties. Most often these other duties consist of safety, quality assurance, support services, or in-patient services.

Medium-sized hospitals (200 to 400 beds) often find it convenient and cost-effective to combine the risk management and quality assurance functions. This also results in well-integrated risk management and quality assurance programs. This approach often does not work well in the larger hospital or those that are self-insured, because of the scope and complexity of the risk management and quality assurance functions in those settings.

A survey conducted by the Association of Hospital Risk Management of New York, Inc. (AHRMNY), in 1988 studied the relationship between hospital size and staffing in various risk management departments. The results of the survey are found in Table 2-1.

Table 2-1 AHRMNY Survey Results

	Hospital Size = Number of Beds				
	26–150	151–300	301–500	501–800	>800
% of risk manager's time devoted to risk management (median)	45%	50%	75%	90%	95%
% with one or more professional asst.	38%	34%	39%	53%	73%
% with two or more professional asst.	19%	11%	17%	33%	45%
% of first asst.'s time devoted to risk management (median)	25%	50%	90%	99%	100%

Source: Risk Management Survey, Association of Hospital Risk Management of New York, Inc., 1988.

What Are the Nature and Complexity of the Institution?

Hospitals offering high-risk services often incur greater losses and require larger risk management departments. High-risk services include obstetrics, emergency/trauma, neonatology, burn units, transplantation units, open heart surgery, orthopedics, neurosurgery, psychiatry, and intensive care. If the facility is a regional referral center and coordinates air/ground transport for any of these services, the liability risk will be even greater.

Teaching hospitals also tend to incur greater losses. In addition to monitoring the appropriate supervision of students, interns, or residents, risk management departments in such institutions must also carefully review and monitor affiliation agreements for liability implications. Therefore, such hospitals usually require larger risk management departments.

What Programs Already Exist in the Hospital That Will Enhance the Risk Management Function?

A hospital with functioning safety, patient/guest relations, and quality assurance programs will have far less work to do in establishing a comprehensive risk management program. A good safety program identifies environmental hazards and prevents injuries to patients, visitors, and staff. An active patient/guest relations program fosters better relationships with patients and is essential to the prevention of litigation. An effective quality assurance program can be of great value in identifying areas of risk and resolving potential liability problems. Therefore, the existence of any of these programs will greatly reduce the amount of work necessary to initiate a comprehensive risk management program.

Does the Hospital Have an Attorney on Staff?

Risk managers often spend a great deal of time dealing with problems involving potential and actual liability. The handling of additional issues such as informed consent, refusal and withdrawal of treatment, confidentiality, patients' rights, and "Do Not Resuscitate" orders are often handled by in-house counsel and can reduce the workload of the risk manager. In hospitals that do not have attorneys on staff, it is often the risk manager who acts as an intermediary between the hospital staff and the outside hospital attorney. However, in hospitals with an attorney on staff, the risk manager spends less time dealing with these issues.

What Are the State's Regulatory Requirements in the Area of Risk Management?

A number of states, including Alaska, Florida, Kansas, Maryland, Massachusetts, New York, North Carolina, Rhode Island, and Washington, have enacted legislation requiring risk management programs in hospitals. These laws often have comprehensive requirements governing risk management, quality assurance, the credentialing process, safety programs, and even the reporting and investigation of certain types of medical incidents by hospitals. The accompanying documentation requirements are most often burdensome. This has resulted in increased staffing needs in affected departments.

ORGANIZATION OF THE RISK MANAGEMENT DEPARTMENT

After analyzing the institution's needs, the administrator or risk manager will have some idea about what the risk manager's responsibilities will be. A comprehensive risk management program includes the following functions:

- Risk control functions
  - —developing, implementing, and maintaining an incident reporting system and other methods of risk identification
  - —investigating and analyzing information generated by risk identification systems and recommending necessary corrective action
  - —providing advice and assistance to hospital and medical staff on matters involving potential liability
  - —reviewing hospital policies and contracts for potential liability exposure and making recommendations for change
  - —educating hospital and medical staff about risk prevention measures
- Risk financing functions
  - —directing and coordinating the hospital's insurance programs
  - —directing and monitoring the handling and defense of the hospital's professional and general liability claims
  - —analyzing and making recommendations to administration and the board on the hospital's risk financing options and decisions
  - —coordinating the functions of the hospital's brokers, consultants, and attorneys
- Administrative functions
  - —directing and supervising the operations of the risk management department

—developing and implementing automated systems for tracking of risk management data

—monitoring compliance with regulatory and Joint Commission requirements

The next question to be decided is to whom the risk manager will report. This is an extremely important decision that will determine the amount of authority the risk manager has. It will also be an indication to the hospital and medical staff about what importance the administration of the hospital attaches to the risk management program. Since the risk manager must interact with a number of hospital departments, and those interactions will often involve recommending policy and procedure changes, the risk manager must have access to administrators who can implement such changes. Thus, the decision of whom the risk manager will report to can have a significant impact on the success of the risk management program.

In its 1988 Risk Management Survey, AHRMNY found that 46.5 percent of the risk managers who responded report to individuals with titles of chief executive officer, administrator, president, or executive director. Nearly all who responded report to someone at the level of vice president or higher.

Decisions will have to be made about which duties the risk manager will have. Will the risk manager be responsible for all risk management functions, including risk financing? (This is usually the case with large, self-insured facilities.) Will the risk manager's responsibilities be limited to risk control functions, with risk financing responsibilities being assigned to a financial officer? (This is often done at smaller, commercially insured hospitals.) Will the risk manager be responsible for workers' compensation, property loss control, or contract review? Will the risk manager have oversight responsibility for other areas, such as quality assurance, safety, credentialing, patient/guest relations, or regulatory compliance?

Of particular importance is the relationship that risk management will have with departments that have related functions, such as safety, quality assurance, patient/guest relations, and credentialing. All of these departments perform risk control functions and generate data that are of mutual interest. Often hospital administrators are concerned with what reporting relationships will result in maximum effectiveness of all of these functions. The size of the institution and the scope of these functions will affect how they are organized. Sometimes the decision is made to merge two or more of these departments. It is important to bear in mind, however, that it is not necessary to merge departments in order to achieve integration. Good communication and mutual committee memberships are often all that is necessary to achieve integration of overlapping functions. Some hospi-

Exhibit 2-1 Sample Job Description—Comprehensive Risk Management Department

---

TITLE: Director of Risk Management

RESPONSIBLE TO: Chief Executive Officer

SUMMARY OF POSITION: Develop, implement, and manage the hospital's risk
management program in accordance with regulatory,
Joint Commission, and institutional requirements

PRIMARY RESPONSIBILITIES:

—Reporting to administration, medical staff, and board of trustees on important
medical/legal issues
—Directing all professional, general, and product liability claims management and
legal defense activities in conjunction with insurance carriers, consultants, and legal
counsel
—Developing, coordinating, and administering hospital-wide systems for risk identification, analysis, and management
—Planning and coordinating risk management educational programs for hospital and
medical staff
—Organizing, managing, and directing the operation of the risk management
department

DETAILED DESCRIPTION OF RESPONSIBILITIES:

Reports immediately to the chief executive officer any serious event involving actual
or potential injury to a patient, visitor, or employee.

Meets biweekly with the chief executive officer and provides detailed reports on all
serious events, claims, and medical/legal issues.

Designs, implements, and maintains a hospital-wide incident reporting system, including an incident investigation system.

Designs, implements, and maintains a direct referral system for the reporting of serious
events by staff.

Develops and maintains appropriate integration with the quality assurance department,
in compliance with regulatory and Joint Commission requirements.

Reports monthly to the Risk Management Committee on serious incidents, claims,
and risk management concerns.

Reports monthly to the Quality Assurance Committee on serious events and risk
management/quality assurance concerns.

Reports monthly to the Safety Committee on incident trends and safety issues.

Attends monthly meetings of the Infection Control Committee.

Directs and coordinates all aspects of insurance management for the institution. This
includes managing self-insurance, excess insurance, and other risk-financing programs
for the hospital.

Prepares materials necessary for renewal of existing insurance policies.

Analyzes existing policies for coverage and exclusion clauses.

Maintains insurance policies and contract files.

Exhibit 2-1 continued

Ensures compliance with state insurance department reporting requirements.

Evaluates correspondence from attorneys, patients, and other outside sources and formulates responses as necessary.

Reports all actual and potential claims to primary and excess carriers as necessary.

Establishes and maintains all legal case files and ensures maximum protection from discoverability.

Directs and coordinates all investigations of actual and potential claims.

Directs all claims-handling and defense preparation activities of the insurance company and defense counsel.

Oversees settlement negotiations. Has independent settlement authority up to $50,000.

Assists defense counsel in preparation of defense strategy and witness selection as necessary.

Assists defense counsel in preparing witnesses for depositions and trials. Provides hospital representation in all liability legal proceedings.

Provides direction and advice as necessary to medical staff on professional liability and medical/legal matters.

Assists clinical chairpersons and department heads in designing risk management programs within their departments.

Directs and conducts educational sessions for medical staff and hospital staff on risk management and component topics.

Renews and revises hospital policies as necessary to maintain adherence to current standards and requirements, and screens for potential liability problems.

Consults with and advises the administrator-on-duty on medical/legal matters. Acts as liaison with hospital counsel.

Reviews contracts, affiliation agreements, leases, construction agreements, and purchase orders as appropriate to evaluate liability exposure.

Develops and maintains risk management profiles on individual physicians and ensures integration of this information into the credentialing process, in compliance with regulatory and Joint Commission requirements.

Directs and coordinates the release of records and information in response to subpoenas, court orders, attorney requests, state investigations, and other inquiries from outside sources.

Consults with and advises the patient representative on the handling of patient complaints.

Directs the automation of incident report data and case file databases.

Maintains risk management statistics and files in compliance with Joint Commission and regulatory requirements. Ensures maximum confidentiality of such information.

Directs the operations of the risk management department and supervises the activities of the risk management professional and clerical/support staff.

tals also resolve this need by having related functions report to the same administrator.

Another important consideration is which committees the risk manager will be a member of. Committee participation not only provides the risk manager with useful information and opportunities to implement risk control measures but is also a reflection of the risk manager's authority within the hospital organization. In addition to the risk management committee, the risk manager should be a member of the quality assurance committee, the safety committee, and the infection control committee. Membership on the other committees may also be desirable, depending upon the organization of the hospital.

Once the scope of the job is defined and the reporting relationships have been determined, a job description can be developed. Exhibit 2-1 presents

Exhibit 2-2 Sample Job Description—Risk Control Program

TITLE: Risk Manager

RESPONSIBLE TO: Associate Administrator, Patient Care Services

SUMMARY OF POSITION: Oversee and monitor the hospital's risk control program

DUTIES AND RESPONSIBILITIES:

Reviews all incident reports and potential liability claims on a daily basis.

Maintains a daily log of all incident reports and potential claims.

Reports all potential claims to insurance carrier and attorney in a timely manner.

Obtains and forwards to insurance carrier and defense attorney any information requested in connection with defense of a lawsuit.

Investigates any serious incidents or potential liability events, and reports findings to insurance carrier and defense attorney.

Consults with hospital attorney regarding any legal questions raised by hospital or medical staff. Acts as liaison between staff and attorney on such matters.

Assists attorney in defense of liability cases by scheduling appointments with hospital staff as requested.

Conducts in-service education sessions with hospital staff as necessary on documentation and related risk management topics.

Reports immediately to associate administrator for patient services any serious incidents or potential liability claims.

Reports monthly to the Quality Assurance/Risk Management Committee on all serious incidents or potential claims and trends of incident report data.

Reports monthly to the Safety Committee on incident report data and trends.

a sample job description for a hospital with a comprehensive risk management program. Exhibit 2-2 shows a sample job description for a hospital in which the risk manager's functions are primarily devoted to risk control. Figures 2-2 and 2-3 show sample tables of organizations.

SALARY AND BUDGET CONSIDERATIONS

Salaries of risk managers vary greatly, depending on the background and responsibilities of the incumbent, the size and nature of the hospital, and the region in which the hospital is located. Recent national data are not available. However, the 1988 AHRMNY survey on risk management did provide some information on salaries in New York State. Again, the salaries seem to be related to hospital size.

Hospital Size # of Beds	Median Annual Salary	% with Annual Salary $46,000
26–150	$31,000	12%
151–300	$35,000	26%
301–500	$36–$40,000	11%
501–800	$46–$50,000	53%
>800	$46–$50,000	64%

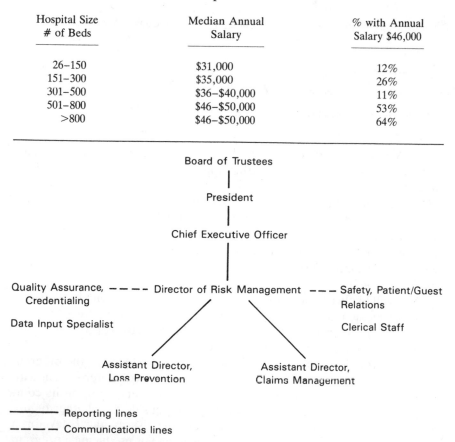

Board of Trustees

President

Chief Executive Officer

Quality Assurance, — — — Director of Risk Management — — — Safety, Patient/Guest
Credentialing   Relations

Data Input Specialist   Clerical Staff

Assistant Director,   Assistant Director,
Loss Prevention   Claims Management

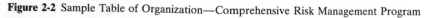

———— Reporting lines

— — — Communications lines

Figure 2-2 Sample Table of Organization—Comprehensive Risk Management Program

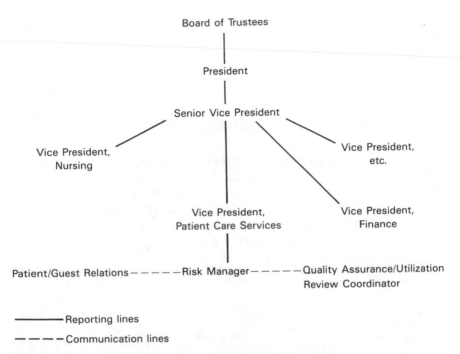

Figure 2-3 Sample Table of Organization—Risk Control Program

The AHRMNY survey also found the median salary for the risk manager's first assistant was $30,000; this appeared to be independent of hospital size.

In determining the salaries to be paid to risk management personnel, the administrator should bear in mind that it will be more advantageous to the institution to offer competitive salaries. Given the confidential nature of the information to be handled by the risk management staff, turnover of staff, particularly clerical and support staff, should be avoided if at all possible.

There will likely be many nonrecurring costs associated with establishing a risk management department. In addition to acquisition of office furniture and supplies, one can anticipate that consultants' fees will be higher the first year that the program is established.

One major expense that will be incurred in the first year of the program is the cost associated with automation. A personal computer system with printer will cost approximately $3,500. Software, depending on its complexity, can cost up to $30,000. One thing to consider is whether or not the hospital has individuals on staff to help the risk manager develop a computer program. This option has the advantage of producing a program tailored to the institution's needs and is much less expensive. There are several commercially available software packages that can be used for this purpose. Many of these cost less than $500 and can produce impressive results. However, developing a program is a time-consuming task requiring a certain amount of technical expertise. Unless the risk manager has had a good amount of experience with computers and has the time to invest in the project, support services from someone trained in automated systems will be required. The hospital may wish to investigate whether engaging a consultant to develop a program using a commercially available package is more cost-effective than purchasing ready-made risk management software.

FINDING THE RIGHT PERSON

Nearly everyone working in the field of risk management today began his or her professional career in another discipline. Because there are no specific training programs for hospital risk management, there is no reliable way of identifying a group of applicants from which to choose. The diversity of backgrounds also makes evaluating an individual's credentials more complicated. Most risk managers today have one or more of the following backgrounds:

Health Care Administration

As the demand for risk managers suddenly increased in the late 1970s and early 1980s, many hospital administrators moved into the field of risk management. These individuals possess the advantage of being extremely well versed in general administrative matters and hospital operations. Individuals with this background are especially suited for risk management positions that have line authority for other hospital departments as well.

Nursing

Nurses also responded to the increased demand for risk management professionals brought on by the liability crisis. Nurses have the advantage of having an intimate knowledge of the delivery of patient care. Their clinical background can also be of great assistance when the evaluation of actual or potential litigation is required. Risk managers with nursing backgrounds generally relate very well to physicians and other hospital staff. This can be an advantage in clinically complex institutions.

Law

Risk managers with legal backgrounds have the advantage of being less dependent on outside counsel, which can result in lower legal fees. Hospitals that have incorporated extensive legal review functions into the risk management position have found it very useful to hire attorneys as risk managers.

Insurance

Risk managers with insurance backgrounds are able to perform claims management activities independently and do not rely as heavily on outside consultants. Again, this can result in considerable savings. Many hospitals with self-insurance programs have found it helpful to have someone with an insurance background on staff in the risk management department.

Medical Records

Individuals with medical records backgrounds are well versed not only in chart reading but also in the intricacies of dealing with attorneys' requests for records and subpoenas.

Finance

Multihospital systems with self-insurance programs often opt for a risk manager with a finance background. These individuals then have risk managers in the member hospitals reporting to them.

There is no one background that is most desirable, although the risk manager needs to have some knowledge of all of the above areas. Any lack of expertise in a particular area can be compensated for by the use of outside consultants and experts or by hiring support staff with the desired background.

Regardless of the background, the individual chosen should possess the following qualities:

Strong Interpersonal Skills

The risk management process works primarily through the actions of the hospital and medical staff. The risk manager needs to be able to communicate effectively with all of these individuals—often regarding very sensitive information—in order to get the job done. A large portion of this process involves "selling" risk management to the staff. Therefore, the successful risk manager is one who can relate well to all levels of hospital staff and who can motivate others to participate in the risk management process.

Management Experience

Although the risk manager is usually a staff person and not a line manager, much of the job involves coordinating the efforts of other hospital departments. Some management experience is desirable for this reason.

Knowledge of the Technical Aspects of Hospital Functions and Health Care

The risk manager will spend considerable time dealing with clinical staff on medical issues. Knowledge of the technical aspects of patient care will make this easier for both the risk manager and the hospital staff.

Risk Management Experience

When starting a risk management department, many decisions about program design will have to be made. Experience in risk management will be essential to these decisions.

Membership in Professional Societies

This is evidence of an individual's commitment to the field of risk management and is especially important because there are no specific training programs for health care risk management. The national society, the American Society for Healthcare Risk Management, confers the designation of Fellow or Diplomat on qualified members. These designations are granted when an individual demonstrates competence and commitment in the field of health care risk management. Such designations are difficult to earn, but membership in the organization is a minimal credential that all risk managers should have.

Evidence of Participation in Continuing Education

Since risk management, like many health care disciplines, is rapidly changing, the risk manager must constantly participate in continuing education to keep knowledge current. Again, the lack of specific training programs for health care risk management makes this an especially important requirement.

Appropriate Educational Background

Although there are no educational programs specific to risk management, some minimum requirements should be sought in a successful candidate. Most risk managers have at least a bachelor's degree, and many have a master's or other advanced degree.

REFERENCES

Association of Hospital Risk Management of New York, Inc. *Risk Management Survey,* 1988 (photocopy).

Brown, B.L. *Risk Management for Hospitals: A Practical Approach.* Rockville, Md.: Aspen Publishers, Inc., 1979.

Kraus, G.P. *Health Care Risk Management: Organization and Claims Administration.* Owings Mills, Md.: Rynd Communications, 1986.

Orlikoff, J.E., and A.M. Vanagunas. *Malpractice Prevention and Liability Control for Hospitals.* Chicago: American Hospital Association, 1981.

Richards, E.P., and K.C. Rathbun. *Medical Risk Management.* Rockville, Md.: Aspen Publishers, Inc., 1983.

Troyer, G.T., and S.L. Salman. *Handbook of Health Care Risk Management.* Rockville, Md.: Aspen Publishers, Inc., 1986.

chapter 3

Gaining Administrative Support for Program Development and Implementation

Josephine Goode-Johnson

A successful risk management program recognizes all elements of loss or risk potential and utilizes a broad range of skills and strategies to avoid, reduce, and eliminate situations that may lead to professional liability claims. Eliciting the cooperation and support of department managers in the risk management process is critical. Segmented risk control responsibilities can inhibit good risk management. In every organization that has achieved an outstanding record of success, it is apparent that senior level and middle management are working together, with responsibility and accountability as common goals. Managers must be educated as to their roles within the risk management process and be held accountable against measurable goals and objectives.

One of the most difficult tasks facing the risk manager is obtaining the cooperation and support of other managers within the organization. Because the risk manager does not have control over department managers, this relationship must be developed and maintained out of mutual respect and understanding of the others' areas of responsibility.

To begin and maintain a successful relationship, there are five equally important areas on which the risk manager should focus:

1. marketing
2. education
3. departmental risk assessment
4. communication and documentation
5. feedback

MARKETING

It is often helpful to schedule a meeting with the department managers to ascertain their current understanding of risk management; determine their departments' needs, goals and objectives; gain an awareness of the day-to-day problems the department managers face; and, most important, to understand the managers' priorities.

This initial meeting will place the risk manager in a better position to determine the approach that will be most effective with a manager, as well as serve as the beginning of a department assessment that will become the foundation of the program. (Individual, department-specific clinical indicators and other assessment tools are found in Chapter 5.)

In marketing the organization's risk management plan to department managers, it is important to begin by establishing common ground. The risk manager should explain that risk management is a management function that incorporates the same skills used in the department manager's job: planning, directing, implementing, controlling, and coordinating activities designed to control loss and maximize program effectiveness.

The goal during this discussion is to develop mutual areas of interest and a mutual support system that will aid in problem identification, assessment, and resolution.

EDUCATION

Once common ground and mutual interest have been established, it is important to share with the department manager those services to be provided by the risk management department that will address many of the department manager's concerns. While risk management programs will vary from institution to institution, some of the basic services most commonly offered to hospital staff include:

- Identification and investigation of
  —potentially compensable events
  —deviations from established policies and procedures
  —potential risk exposure
- Medical-legal reference service
  —policy and procedure development
  —referral to appropriate parties, policies, and procedures
  —medical record documentation
  —legal liaison

- Defense coordination
  —what to do in the event of a claim, suit, or attorney contact
  —how to discuss adverse occurrences with patients and families
  —litigation management
  —insurance compliance and notification
- System coordination
  —movement of stagnated issues through the system toward resolution
  —preparation of interdisciplinary reports containing information gathered by the risk management department that can assist other departments with program development

The risk manager should also use this opportunity to alleviate some of the manager's anxieties regarding territory, the usurpation of authority, and the possibility of the risk manager's getting involved without the department manager's awareness. It is important to emphasize that risk management will coordinate with and support the manager's role, not compete with it. Inform the manager how information is collected and analyzed and how and in what form the information will be made available to the manager to aid in program development.

DEPARTMENTAL RISK ASSESSMENT

In the current competitive health environment, department managers must understand that the objectives of risk management are to protect, in an effective, economical way, the assets of the institution from a single catastrophic loss or from an accumulation of losses that could significantly affect its financial stability. It should also be emphasized that a second goal is to promote and guarantee quality patient care.

In assessing the department's potentially high-risk activities, the risk manager should consider the following:

- Manager's overall understanding of the institution's goals and objectives
- Current departmental structures in place (i.e., committees, reporting relationships, department organization); whether interdisciplinary committees (i.e., emergency department, trauma, surgery, intensive care, obstetrics, neonatology, pediatrics) meet when appropriate
- Policies, procedures, and standards currently in place; whether old policies are kept

- Methods used to disseminate information within the department (i.e., staff meetings, shift reports, communication logs, memorandums)
- Methods used to increase communication and motivation of staff
- Resources and backups
- Potential for integrating problems within existing institution's structures (i.e., manager's awareness of committee structure and function)
- Accountability and reporting structure
- Interactions between manager and staff
- Manager's awareness of quality assurance and risk management techniques
- Incident and claim reporting system; department's understanding and compliance with it
- Manager's areas and scope of responsibility
- Willingness to support risk management functions
- Employee grievance system
- Patient complaint system
- High-risk areas (to be analyzed in greater detail during second meeting)
- Staffing patterns in relation to services provided
- Methods of documentation
- Equipment, property, policies, and procedures
- Safety awareness (i.e., awareness of policies and protocols)
- Services offered within area
- Security of patient information
- Supervision of staff; orientation and training
  —skills inventory
  —documentation of additional training
  —credential verification
- Medical supplies and equipment
  —prepurchase evaluation
  —pretesting
  —system for sequestering defective equipment
  —product recall system
  —preventive maintenance programs
- Safety and health
  —employee accident prevention
  —occupational exposures
  —right-to-know policies
  —environmental hazards

- Security
  —pharmacy
  —patient valuables
  —confidentiality

Following the initial assessment, a second meeting should be scheduled to discuss specifics of the risk management program's functions and services and to lay the foundation for the department manager's involvement in this process. At this point, assessments of department-specific clinical indicators, such as those described in Chapter 5, can be performed.

Departmental Responsibilities

Like any management function, risk management must be performed in a systematic and continuous manner. Such an approach further helps the risk manager recognize exposures, judge the frequency of loss, and determine potential dollar loss figures in preparation for loss prevention and risk financing activities.

Loss avoidance is obviously the ideal goal to strive for, but a goal virtually impossible to attain. With increased technology and an increasingly sophisticated medical environment, perfection is difficult to achieve. Unfortunately, perfection is what the consumer has come to expect! To achieve maximum loss avoidance potential, risk management must carefully analyze practice and strive to assist clinicians in providing service of the maximum possible quality. When total loss avoidance is impossible, the risk manager and department managers must then practice other techniques to minimize the financial risk to the hospital. The department manager is essential in exercising loss control techniques. Because every aspect of rendering care contains an element of risk, decisions regarding the department's performance should include the probability and severity of losses that could occur. These determinations must then be carefully evaluated in an attempt to minimize the potential of patient harm and hospital risk. The department manager should be advised that decisions regarding mergers, acquisitions, hold-harmless contracts, and agreements and other techniques for minimizing or transferring risk can be employed to limit the hospital's financial exposure. The risk manager must emphasize that timely notice is imperative in implementing any loss avoidance or transfer technique.

Department managers should also be advised that risks can be transferred or assumed by others by contractual agreements. Consequently, they should be made aware that contractual relationships should be formalized by written agreements to avoid unnecessary and undesirable assumptions of liability and to clearly outline the responsibilities of both parties. Additionally, contractual agreements should be reviewed carefully by risk management and legal counsel, as applicable, prior to signing. Timely review allows appropriate transfer of responsibility and assessment of risk management and insurance exposures.

Loss control can be divided into two areas: loss prevention and loss reduction. Loss prevention involves controlling the frequency of losses (e.g., an education program on how to avoid back injury while lifting patients). The department manager can practice loss control through safety rules, regulations, and training programs that are designed to reduce injuries to patients, visitors, and employees.

Loss reduction techniques are designed to minimize the overall size of losses. For example, installation of fire walls reduces overall damage caused by fire. Disaster plans also reduce damage to property, employees, patients, and visitors. Effective loss control through the use of safety and risk management committees will also have a direct impact on future risk management costs.

The risk manager and department manager should establish a time to discuss claims (open and closed), to keep the manager informed and aid in gauging the effectiveness of the loss control program. The risk manager also may offer to assist in safety inspections and provide staff education and information updates.

Other loss control techniques that should be discussed with the department manager in this context include

- incident reporting
- disaster activities
- patient complaint activities
- preventive maintenance activities
- contract review
- product recall and purchasing
- use of patient safety and restraining devices
- confidentiality procedures
- experimental treatment programs
- patient valuables storage
- documentation standards
- committee functions
- staff selection and supervision
- orientation and continuing education training programs

- patient admitting and identification procedures
- standards, policies, and procedures
- training programs
- premises and equipment inspection and maintenance procedures
- employee supervision

COMMUNICATION/DOCUMENTATION/FEEDBACK

It is imperative that regularly scheduled meeting times be established to discuss the program and the achievement of goals and objectives. This relationship will provide the department manager with the necessary information, awareness, and administrative support to make informed decisions that will have a positive impact on the institution's policies, products, and services. Feedback to staff, reflecting their participation in the risk management process, is also critical and will enable staff to see the substantial benefits that can be achieved through the process. Meetings also permit the risk manager to determine and take the necessary steps to eliminate and reduce risks, identify new problem areas, and maintain a feedback loop.

Additionally, communication can be enhanced between risk management and operational departments through the use of a risk management manual. This manual may be broad or focused in scope, but it should include as much of the following information as applicable. The manual should be reviewed and updated regularly, and staff should be encouraged to assist in this process and, if appropriate, to tailor policies to meet department-specific needs. At least the following should be included in a manual:

- a management policy statement that affirms and supports the risk management process
- an organizational chart delineating reporting relationships
- descriptions of the institution's retention/insurance program, in simple language
- incident and claims reporting procedures and sample forms
- a schedule of educational programs offered by the risk management department
- the patient complaint system, with emergency contact names and numbers
- common consent issues and answers

- guidelines for contract review
- reporting mechanisms for relevant medical staff committees relating to risk management
- important telephone numbers and ways to contact the risk manager in case of an emergency
- medical record policies related to risk management

COMMUNICATION

A fundamental goal of both the department and the risk managers should be to improve employee awareness of risk management and to practice safety, out of concern and respect for the patient. Employees must be motivated to remain attuned to patient attitudes, perceptions, and expectations, as well as to be alert to the possibility of patient dissatisfaction. It should be emphasized that the employees' risk management role is as significant as their other assigned duties and that compliance with risk management goals is expected and will provide increasing benefits to both the patient and the staff.

CONCLUSION

Before a program can operate effectively, there must be commitment to risk management from all levels within the institution. It is critical that managers recognize their legal and moral responsibilities to provide quality care, to identify the inherent risks associated with providing that care, and to minimize loss effectively.

By actively soliciting and supporting their efforts, risk managers will achieve greater loss control from department managers, encourage a higher priority level and acceptance for risk management functions, and significantly reduce the probability of unexpected liability claims.

PART II

Assessing the Needs of the Institution

These chapters in Part II will provide readers with information necessary to analyze the clinical risk areas within their institutions and to develop monitors and department-specific clinical indicators to assess those risks. Clearly, it is the clinical risks that will in the long run have the greatest impact on the financial integrity of the institution; their successful management will guarantee that the highest possible quality of care is rendered.

The inclusion of specific "monitors" will also assist in sensitizing the risk manager and department staff to aspects of their clinical practice that need continual monitoring. Although they have been provided only for the high-risk areas, their format can easily be adapted for other areas.

chapter 4

Risk Identification Strategies in Hospitals

Elizabeth A. Lee

Since the mid-1970s the number of claims and lawsuits against physicians, hospitals, and other providers of health care has increased dramatically. With this rise in malpractice claims alleging negligence as the cause of the adverse patient outcomes, health care institutions have taken an increased interest in controlling their clinical risk exposures. The field of health care risk management has developed into a critical tool for preventing and managing liability exposures, for improving the quality of patient care, and for protecting the financial assets of health care institutions.

Risk management has been defined as the process of "planning, organizing, leading, and controlling the activities of the organization in order to minimize the adverse effects of accidental losses on that organization at reasonable cost."[1]

In order to control risks, G.L. Head and S. Horn, II, suggest such techniques as risk avoidance, loss prevention, and loss reduction. Risk avoidance involves eliminating all losses associated with a particular activity, loss prevention involves reducing the chance that a mishap will occur, and loss reduction emphasizes reducing the severity and impact of losses once they occur.[2]

Because of the nature of current medical interventions, complete risk avoidance is not feasible in health care organizations. Therefore, loss reduction and loss prevention should be the areas of emphasis in hospital risk management. Loss reduction techniques are commonly employed in current methods of claims management, whereby administrative, legal, and clinical personnel seek to contain losses resulting from negligent or potentially negligent actions of employees or associated medical staff members. (These claims management techniques will be discussed in Chapter 6.)

Loss prevention techniques focus on reducing the frequency of occurrences likely to result in claims and/or lawsuits. In order to prevent potentially compensable events, it is necessary to identify the various exposures to risk existing in various health care disciplines and settings. After identifying the potential areas of risk (through surveys, incident trend analysis, and other methods), actions can be taken to modify risky circumstances or behaviors.

This chapter will provide a method for evaluating the existing strategies for risk identification within individual institutions and will suggest options for establishing a system that will meet the requirements of accreditation standards.

ASSESSMENT OF EXISTING INSTITUTIONAL PROGRAMS

Evaluating a health care organization's risk prevention activities requires an examination of (1) the structure of the risk management department, (2) the data management activities of the staff, and (3) the degree of the risk management department's integration with other hospital departments involved in monitoring the quality of patient care. This assessment requires an inquiry that reaches beyond traditional risk management activities to evaluate risk identification efforts existing throughout the institution.

Structure of the Risk Management Department

The issues related to structure of the risk management office include an examination of the roles of various staff members. Several questions are relevant:

- Is there one risk manager who handles claims management as well as prevention activities?
- Is there in-house counsel?
- Are other quality assurance activities performed by the office?

If one individual is responsible for claims management activities, prevention activities often take a reactive rather than a proactive posture. Although there will always be unexpected incidents requiring subsequent changes in practice or policy, it is important to try to identify risk exposures before claims or lawsuits emerge. Larger institutions, self-insured for professional liability and with in-house counsel, may find it desirable to separate the functions of claims management and loss prevention between two risk managers. Institutions that lack in-house counsel and are not self-insured may concentrate their efforts on early risk identification and loss prevention, if all claims are managed primarily by the outside insurance company.

Data Management Activities

Another component of a hospital's self-assessment is an evaluation of the types of data collected and analyzed in the effort to control risk exposures. The incident report is a central tool, used for both claims management and loss prevention activities. All occurrences resulting in actual or potential injury to the patient or that may lead to a claim or lawsuit should be reported to the risk management office. To ensure the completeness of reporting by health care providers, it is imperative to enhance reporting patterns through education of personnel and through efforts to streamline the reporting process for the convenience of practitioners. In addition to standard written reports, health care providers should be encouraged to call the office directly and/or to call a telephone answering service. Whether or not the incident reporting system is computerized, identification of trends and clusters of events is central to a loss prevention program.

In addition to incident report data, information from surveys and inspections can be used to identify the clinical risk exposure of individual departments. Such surveys and the data from quality improvement efforts (which use clinical indicators to identify potential or actual problems with care) provide valuable information for risk identification. These additional methods are described fully in Chapter 5, which addresses the evaluation of high-risk specialty areas.

Interaction with Other Departments

One organizational issue concerns whether the risk management department is housed separately or with quality assurance or patient/guest relations. Some hospitals have one person performing the functions of more than one office. Other institutions split these activities between departments or personnel. Whenever possible, the risk management office should be organized to permit it access to incident data and to indicators of quality problems generated from other offices or departments.

The interaction may be accomplished by different means. If more than one office is responsible for quality assurance and risk management functions, the personnel could be accountable to the same senior-level manager. Alternatively, the reporting channels could remain separate, but the information systems used by risk management and quality assurance could be linked so that critical problems with patient care may be shared readily. Computer programs can also be developed to allow for the sharing of appropriate information among departments.

Additionally, the activities of clinical departments and medical staff committees should be examined to determine what types of quality assurance functions are currently in place to guard against high-risk practices. If individual departments are performing morbidity and mortality reviews, the minutes from these conferences may provide valuable information related to problem practices. The minutes of medical staff committees that review infection control practices, safety programs, transfusion patterns, and specialized areas of clinical practice should also assist in identifying high-risk areas and high-risk practices. In some cases, it may be necessary to merge the activities of two or more committees in order to eliminate duplication and to centralize reporting efforts, though care must be taken to avoid the loss of protection afforded under state peer review laws. Whatever the committee structure, medical staff members should be responsible for overseeing the actions of the quality assurance and risk management functions as they relate to the clinical practices of physicians.

INTEGRATION OF RISK MANAGEMENT AND QUALITY ASSURANCE: THE "AGENDA FOR CHANGE"

As mentioned earlier, the ability of the risk manager to collect and analyze data represents the central strength of a successful loss prevention program. Integration of risk management activities with those of quality assurance departments has become a popular method of identifying risks. With recent changes made in the activities of quality assurance departments, aimed at meeting the revised accreditation standards outlined in the 1986 Joint Commission on Accreditation of Healthcare Organizations (Joint Commission) "Agenda for Change," risk management functions have become more closely linked with quality improvement efforts.

Methods of evaluating quality of health care can be classified into three general categories, as described by Avedis Donabedian: structure, process, and outcome. Assessment of structure involves the evaluation of facilities and the capabilities of personnel. Evaluation of process involves determination of the most appropriate means to affect change. Evaluation of outcomes assesses the end results of health care.[3]

Historically, the Joint Commission, a voluntary accreditation organization, measured only structure and process indicators of quality. In recent years, however, there has been an increasing emphasis in the literature on using outcome measures to indicate the quality of antecedent care.[4] As a result of this shift in theoretical premise, the Joint Commission has set the stage for a new level of quality assessment in health care delivery. At its December 10, 1988, meeting, the Joint Commission Board of Commissioners approved an official definition of quality patient care: "the degree to which patient care services increase the probability of desired patient outcomes and reduce the probability of undesired outcomes, given the current state of knowledge."[5] This definition of quality reflects the focus of loss prevention activities within the risk management framework.

The "Agenda for Change" was announced in 1986 by Dennis S. O'Leary, M.D., President of the Joint Commission. As a major part of this change in focus, the Joint Commission projects that by 1992 it will have in place a new system for evaluation upon which to base its accreditation guidelines. The new standards will emphasize data-driven quality assurance and will include measures of organizational as well as clinical performance.

The measures of organizational performance will evaluate the manner in which the institution supports the process of quality assurance, as well as management characteristics and decisions influencing the provision of care. These measures focus on a system-wide commitment to improvement through ongoing assessment by objective indicators, and they emphasize problem resolution as necessary.

According to Dr. O'Leary, the institution of this new evaluation method will require a "professional culture change" at both the organizational and clinical levels, which will give incentives for identifying problems and then taking action to correct them.[6] At the heart of the development of the new clinical evaluation method is the identification of specific clinical indicators. The Joint Commission is currently working with practitioners to distill, from the hundreds of possible indicators, the most telling measures of performance. However, the Joint Commission expects hospitals and practitioners to develop individualized measures of quality, to be supplemented by those recommended by the expert panels. According to the Joint Commission, these indicators are not meant to depict directly the quality of clinical performance: "Rather, they are a means of predictably raising sound questions about the quality of care. Indicators are 'flags' or 'screens' which highlight the need for problem analysis and peer review as appropriate."[7]

The Joint Commission expects that hospitals will develop systematic, objective methods for identifying potential problems with care and for initiating actions to correct these problems. Furthermore, Joint Commission standards require that physician-specific information related to quality assurance and liability experience be used in the process of credentialing and reappointment.

In addition to these new standards for quality assurance, the Joint Commission has developed standards for the review of risk management programs, which emphasize the importance of loss prevention activities. These new standards were effective January 1, 1989, and require that institutions have methods for identifying areas of potential risk and for intervening for the purpose of reducing risk in the "clinical aspects of patient care and safety." In order to achieve these goals, hospitals must show "operational linkages" between risk management and quality assurance functions.[8]

A Model for Integration

In light of these efforts to improve quality and to meet the requirements of accreditation, hospitals must begin to grapple with difficult questions:

- How should a quality assurance/risk management program be structured?
- Who will be in charge of supervising personnel?
- Where should it be placed in an organizational framework?
- How will the various components of risk management quality assurance and utilization review interact with and report to one another?
- What types of data will be collected, analyzed, and reported?
- What type of computerized system (hardware and software) will be necessary to support data collection efforts?
- How will the data generated by such a system be protected from discovery by outside parties?
- What changes should be made within the medical staff committee structure to facilitate reporting and accountability and to reduce the incidence of duplication?

These decisions must be made within individual institutions, since each organization has different priorities and a different structure. One example of how programs within a hospital can be integrated for the common purpose of improving quality of patient care is demonstrated by the model in Figure 4-1.

This model depicts an effort to achieve operational linkages between quality assurance and risk management and also complies with Joint Commission standards and the demands of third party payors for quality ac-

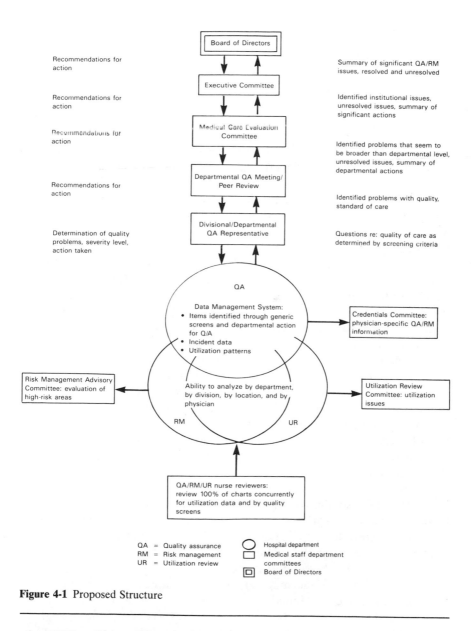

Figure 4-1 Proposed Structure

countability. The model is based on a centralized database for information pertaining to issues of quality care. Care review nurses screen charts for predetermined indicators of quality (to include both generic and department-specific criteria), as well as for utilization data and potentially compensable events. Significant findings are entered into the database and sent to the risk management office so that events requiring investigation and claims coordination may be identified.

Potential quality of care problems are then sent to the appropriate physician quality assurance representative or nursing coordinator for review. In addition to the medical record-generated clinical screens, any risk management incident reports identifying potential quality of care problems are entered into the system for appropriate review by the departments. This objective system provides the information necessary for systematic quality assurance, utilization review, credentialing, and reappointment, as well as for meaningful loss prevention activities.

In addition to their current activities of reviewing risk management data, infection control statistics, blood use data, drug use data, and surgical case indicators, clinical departments within a hospital must establish means for reviewing individual cases identified by predetermined clinical indicators of quality. These efforts of criteria-based review should derive from an understanding by the medical staff of the central tenets of quality assurance, which are to identify problem areas in clinical practice and to take action toward their resolution. If a review by the quality assurance representative identifies a problem with the care rendered, the case should be taken to the departmental quality assurance meeting for review and recommendation for action.

If an issue cannot be resolved by the department, it should be taken to the hospital's quality review committee, the executive committee, and ultimately, the board of directors for determination of any action to be taken. Potentially compensable events would always be referred to risk management for claims management action. In addition, summary data and trend analysis would be reported to the oversight medical staff committees and the board of directors.

This process requires the commitment and involvement of both the medical staff and the administration of the hospital. Although peer review must be performed by similarly credentialed providers, the institution must provide the structure to support these activities. As hospitals make decisions related to organizational structure, committee responsibilities, and computerization needs, the support of administrators as well as medical staff members is of paramount importance. Furthermore, it is imperative that decisions that affect the functions of more than one hospital department be coordinated jointly. For integration to be successful, some programs may need to be merged or eliminated to prevent duplication of effort and to promote the efficient use of resources.

NOTES

1. G.L. Head and S. Horn II, *Essentials of the Risk Management Process*, vol. 1 (Malvern, Penn.: Insurance Institute of America, 1985), p. 6.

2. Ibid, p. 17.

3. A. Donabedian, "Evaluating the Quality of Medical Care," *Milbank Memorial Fund Quarterly* 44 (1966): 166–206.

4. A. Donabedian, "The Quality of Medical Care," in *Quality Assurance in Hospitals: Strategies for Assessment and Implementation,* N.O. Graham, ed. (Rockville, Md.: Aspen Publishers, Inc., 1982), pp. 15–34.

5. "JCAHO Adopts Definition of Quality Patient Care," *Modern Healthcare* 18 (December 16, 1988).

6. D.S. O'Leary, NCMH Managers' Forum Lecture, delivered at Chapel Hill, N.C., Dec. 9, 1987.

7. Joint Commission on Accreditation of Hospitals, *The Joint Commission's Agenda for Change.* 1986 (Statement paper), p. 4.

8. The Joint Commission on Accreditation of Healthcare Organizations, *Accreditation Manual for Hospitals, 1989* (Chicago: Joint Commission on Accreditation of Healthcare Organizations, 1989).

chapter 5

Evaluating High-Risk Specialty Areas

Elizabeth A. Lee

The previous chapter emphasized the importance of assessing the needs of an institution as they relate to the process of risk prevention. Criteria for evaluating the institution with regard to departmental structure, data collection, and integration with other hospital departments were outlined. This chapter will elaborate on methods for utilizing data to systematically identify high-risk areas and to take actions to reduce risks in the clinical aspects of patient care.

Hospital loss prevention programs may be structured in varied ways, depending upon the organizational framework of the institution, the method of liability insurance coverage, and the existing departments involved with risk assessment. However, in order to be successful in identifying potential risks in clinical practice, the following components must exist:

1. a method to conduct interviews, chart reviews, and inspections of individual departments to identify safety hazards as well as risk exposures in clinical care
2. the ability to identify trends and clusters of incidents reported to the risk management department
3. the integration of risk management information with other sources of data designed to identify problems with medical care, such as quality improvement efforts based on review by clinical indicators

These three sources of information may then be combined to present a total picture of risk exposure within a department. The findings of departmental reviews may be compared to national standards of care published by professional societies, the Joint Commission on Accreditation of Healthcare Organizations (Joint Commission), or condensed from verdicts and settlements in malpractice cases. Once the known high-risk areas of a

51

specialty are outlined, actions can be taken to correct deficient practices and to establish means of monitoring patient outcomes.

This type of process may be said to integrate the structure, process, and outcome methods for measuring quality. The hospital may identify general and departmental problems related to structure and process through the process of surveying departments. Then, incident reports and department-specific clinical indicator screens can be used to measure outcomes of care.

DEPARTMENTAL SURVEYS

The purpose of departmental risk assessment surveys is to attempt to identify deficiencies in the quality of care as they relate to known areas of risk. A survey consists of chart reviews, inspections of patient care areas, and interviews with selected physicians and nurses. Examples of risk assessment forms for chart reviews and inspections are seen in Exhibits 5-1 through 5-6. General information can be supplemented by specific items related to the specialty. For example, in reviews of obstetric charts, it is important to note whether or not the fetal heart rate was consistently documented in relation to uterine contractions and oxytocin administration.

CHART REVIEWS

The chart review segment of the risk assessment survey enables the risk manager to evaluate the quality of chart documentation, the completeness of records, and the evidence of provider involvement with care (Exhibits 5-1 through 5-3). In addition, one is able to examine the level of attending physician supervision over students and residents. Since the medical record is generally the most important piece of evidence in a medical malpractice action, it is imperative that the risk manager evaluate each department's standard for documentation.

INSPECTIONS OF PATIENT CARE AREAS

The aim of clinic and unit inspections is to identify obvious physical safety hazards, noncompliance with known standards of practice, and methods established for such things as medication distribution and monitoring of patients. Although the inspection must be adapted to meet the needs of the specialty, the examples provided in Exhibits 5-4 and 5-5 generally address institutional concerns.

Exhibit 5-1 Ambulatory Care Risk Assessment Survey—Chart Review Form

CHART REVIEW FORM

Person completing review: _____ Location: _____

Date: _____ Form #: _____

1. Is there a statement about allergies and/or sensitivities written on the front of the patient's chart or on the first page?

   a. _____ Yes　b. _____ No

2. Are progress notes and/or clinic visit notes in chronological order in the patient's chart?

   a. _____ Yes　b. _____ No

3. Is there a completed Medical Records Summary Sheet at the front of the patient's chart, which outlines the significant diagnoses, medications, and procedures in the patient's medical history?

   a. _____ Complete　b. _____ Incomplete

   IF INCOMPLETE, SPECIFY MISSING INFORMATION: _____

   _____

   _____

4. Are entries in the chart generally legible or illegible?

   a. _____ Legible　b. _____ Illegible

5. Are entries in the chart written in black or blue ink?

   a. _____ Black ink

   b. _____ Blue ink

   c. _____ Other

6. Are vital signs noted at the time of the last clinic visit? (Check all that apply)

   a. _____ Weight

   b. _____ Temperature

   c. _____ Blood Pressure

   d. _____ Other: _____

7. Within the last three visits, is there documentation of patient education regarding medications, home care, etc.?

   a. _____ Yes　b. _____ No

8. For the last three clinic visits, are clinical findings clearly specified?

   a. _____ Yes　b. _____ No

9. For the last three visits, is a diagnostic impression clearly specified?

   a. _____ Yes　b. _____ No

10. Are medication and other therapeutic orders or changes clearly specified for the last three visits?

    a. _____ Yes　b. _____ No

11. Is there a signed informed consent form for each procedure documented on the Medical Records Summary Sheet?

    a. _____ Yes　b. _____ No

12. Is there an up-to-date history and physical (i.e., within the last year)?

    a. _____ Yes　b. _____ No

13. Are the name of the referring physician and the reason for the referral documented? (See first clinic visit note)

    a. _____ Yes　b. _____ No

Exhibit 5-2 In-Patient Risk Assessment Survey—Chart Review Form

CHART REVIEW FORM

Person completing form: _____ Location: _____

Date: _____ Form #: _____

1. Was a statement about allergies and/or sensitivities written in the chart at the time of admission?

   a. _____ Yes   b. _____ No

2. Was a complete history and physical performed at the time of admission?

   a. _____ Yes   b. _____ No

3. Were the name of the referring physician and the reason for referral documented at the time of admission?

   a. _____ Yes   b. _____ No

4. Was a statement written at the time of admission to the unit about patient's current medications?

   a. _____ Yes   b. _____ No

5. For each progress note in the past three days, are the clinical impressions clearly specified?

   a. _____ Yes   b. _____ No

6. For each progress note in the past three days, is a plan of treatment clearly specified?

   a. _____ Yes   b. _____ No

7. Is there a progress note written by the attending physician at least every other day?

   a. _____ Yes   b. _____ No

8. Are there cosignatures by the attending physician on all medical student notes?

   a. _____ Yes   b. _____ No

9. Is there a signed informed consent form for each procedure documented for the admission?

   a. _____ Yes   b. _____ No

10. If the procedure required general anesthesia, is there an additional note by the anesthesiologist documenting informed consent for the anesthesia?

    a. _____ Yes   b. _____ No

    IF YES, DOES THAT NOTE CONTAIN DOCUMENTATION OF THE PATIENT'S DENTAL HEALTH STATUS?

    a. _____ Yes   b. _____ No

11. Do medication orders on admission and for the past three days contain the following information:

    a. Route?   _____ % Yes   _____ % No
    b. Dosage?   _____ % Yes   _____ % No
    c. Frequency? _____ % Yes   _____ % No

12. For the past three days, do the nursing notes document the reasons for and effects from prn medication?

    a. _____ Yes   b. _____ No

13. Do the nursing notes for the last three days document the following information with regard to the administration of medications:

    a. Time given?   _____ Yes   _____ No
    b. Route of administration? _____ Yes   _____ No
    c. Dosage?   _____ Yes   _____ No

Exhibit 5-2 continued

> d. Signatures of nurses? _____ Yes _____ No
> 14. Was the patient's weight recorded at the time of admission?
>   a. _____ Yes b. _____ No
> 15. For the past three days, do the nursing notes document vital signs and blood pressure as frequently as indicated in the medical orders (at least once per day)?
>   a. _____ Yes b, _____ No
> 16. Are nursing focus notes written in the progress note section?
>   a. _____ Yes b. _____ No
> 17. Indicate which of the following sections of the medical record are in chronological order and dated?
>   a. _____ Progress notes
>   b. _____ Nursing notes
>   c. _____ Orders
> 18. Are entries in the chart generally legible or illegible?
>   a. _____ Legible b. _____ Illegible
> 19. Are all pages of the chart stamped with the patient's name, date of birth, and medical record number?
>   a. _____ Yes b. _____ No
> 20. Are entries in the chart written in black or blue ink?
>   a. _____ Black ink
>   b. _____ Blue ink
>   c. _____ Other

PROVIDER INTERVIEWS

Interviews with physicians and nurses serve to heighten their awareness of high-risk areas within their specialties and of the issues most frequently giving rise to the establishment of negligence in malpractice cases. In addition, these conversations allow the risk manager to determine whether existing policies and procedures conform to national standards or known safety practices. (See Exhibit 5-6.)

Information from clinical specialty journals and literature providing information about malpractice verdicts are used to define the standards of care within a specialty, as well as its known areas of risk. Historical trend information for various departments also will help to more clearly identify specific individual institutional risks. After the areas of risk are determined, questions for physician interviews and items for chart reviews and inspections may be articulated, and appropriate monitors may be developed.

TRENDING OF INCIDENT REPORTS

Another important method for identifying potential and actual areas of risk is through the examination of incident trends. In addition to tracking

Exhibit 5-3 Anesthesiology Risk Assessment

CHART REVIEW FORM

Location: _____

Date of Surgery _____/_____/_____   Date of Review _____/_____/_____

1. Preoperative assessment—were the following items present in the note:
   a. Patient's medical and surgical history
      Yes _____ No _____
   b. Current medications
      Yes _____ No _____
   c. Allergies
      Yes _____ No _____
   d. Dental health status
      Yes _____ No _____
   e. Vital signs (BP, Pulse, RR, Temp)
      Yes _____ No _____
   f. Significant lab values
      Yes _____ No _____
   g. Physical assessment by anesthesiologist
      —cardiovascular Yes _____ No _____
      —pulmonary   Yes _____ No _____
      —neurological   Yes _____ No _____
   h. Order for premedication
      Yes _____ No _____
   i. NPO/diet status
      Yes _____ No _____
   j. Attending note/signature
      Yes _____ No _____
2. Intraoperative anesthesia record—was it complete with:
   a. q 5 min BP and pulse and q 15 min ECG reading, temp, pulse ox, ET CO_2, F_1O_2, vent settings, controlled vs. spontaneous respirations?
      Yes _____ No _____
      (Circle missing items)
   b. Was there documentation of intubation with type of ETT used and whether or not it was cuffed?
      Yes _____ No _____
   c. Are significant events numbered and fully explained?
      Yes _____ No _____
   d. Was there an attending note and signature?
      Yes _____ No _____
   e. Were intake and output documented?
      TF = _____
   f. Was the time of discharge to RR documented?
      Yes _____ No _____
3. Postoperative assessment:
   a. Was an immediate post-op note written in the PACU?
      Yes _____ No _____
   b. Did an anesthesiologist write the note to d/c from the PACU?
      Yes _____ No _____
   c. Was there a note written from a postoperative anesthesia visit?
      Yes _____ No _____

falls and medication errors throughout the hospital, it is imperative that the risk manager understand the areas of risk potential within various medical specialties and have the ability to track patterns of relevant events. For example, data related to specific types of surgical procedure complications resulting in adverse patient outcomes are critical in assessing the relative risk for liability within the department of surgery.

Many hospitals are beginning to track incident report data with a computerized system. In such a system, incidents may be classified according to the type of occurrence, the location of the event, the department involved, the staff member(s) involved, and the type of claim made, if applicable. This type of system is extremely beneficial in the tracking of events over time. Departments should be supplied with summary information monthly so that the patterns of occurrences may be evaluated during the quality review process.

QUALITY SCREENS

Finally, the data generated from quality improvement efforts, which include reviews of generic and department-specific screens, may be used to identify risk areas. Some institutions choose to merge this data with the information from incident reports. Generic quality screens, such as those used by the Health Care Financing Administration to evaluate Medicare cases, can be supplemented with department-specific clinical indicators.[1]

Medical records should also be systematically screened for generic and specific indicators in order to highlight potential quality problems. Once the records are screened, the data can be entered into a review process similar to the model described in the previous chapter. As outlined in the description of the model, review of potential quality problems must be conducted by similarly credentialed practitioners.

The data obtained from quality screens can also be combined with incident report data reflecting similar occurrences, to obtain complete trending information. A system for peer review should be established such that adverse events are evaluated in the context of the total number of patients seen or procedures performed. Without adequate denominator data, numbers of complications or deaths have little meaning.

EVALUATION OF HIGH-RISK DISCIPLINES

The following examples demonstrate the process for identifying risk and evaluating a department's exposures to loss. In every review, the general risk assessment principles should be evaluated so that institution-wide is-

Exhibit 5-4 Ambulatory Care Risk Assessment Survey—Clinic Inspection Form

---

CLINIC INSPECTION FORM

Person completing form: _____ Date: _____
Location: _____
Time: _____

Patient waiting area:
1. Are there toys available (Pediatrics, Fam. Med., OB, Surgery)?
   a. _____ Yes   b. _____ No
2. Can conversations among health care personnel or between health care personnel and patients be overheard from waiting area?
   a. _____ Yes   b. _____ No
3. Is there a means to communicate privately with the clerk regarding billing and/ or appointment information?
   a. _____ Yes   b. _____ No

Readiness for emergencies:
1. Is the emergency cart located such that it is convenient to all patient care areas?
   a. _____ Yes   b. _____ No
2. Is the lock on the emergency cart intact?
   a. _____ Yes   b. _____ No
3. Indicate which emergency care items are located in the clinic:
   a. _____ Emergency oxygen tank and tubing
   b. _____ Appropriate intubation trays (pediatric or adult)
   c. _____ Ambu bag
   d. _____ Face masks
   e. _____ Electrocardiograph machine (EKG)
   f. _____ Defibrillator
4. Is there a procedure room in the clinic for invasive procedures?
   a. _____ Yes   b. _____ No
5. Is a supply of IV fluids and lines available in the clinic?
   a. _____ Yes   b. _____ No

Medication control:
1. Are prescription pads kept out of sight of patients?
   a. _____ Yes   b. _____ No
2. Are syringes kept out of sight of patients?
   a. _____ Yes   b. _____ No
3. Are medications kept out of sight of patients?
   a. _____ Yes   b. _____ No
4. Is there a locked narcotics cabinet in the clinic?
   a. _____ Yes   b. _____ No
5. Is there an up-to-date narcotics record used for signing out controlled medications?
   a. _____ Yes   b. _____ No
6. Are the narcotics counted daily by an RN and one other health care provider?
   a. _____ Yes   b. _____ No
7. Are there sealed receptacles for disposal of syringes and needles in every exam room?
   a. _____ Yes   b. _____ No

Exhibit 5-4 continued

General:
1. Do all employees wear name tags?
   a. _____ Yes b. _____ No
2. Can the patient bathrooms be locked from the inside?
   a. _____ Yes b. _____ No
   IF YES, DOES THE STAFF HAVE A KEY TO OPEN THEM WHEN
   NECESSARY?
   a. _____ Yes b. _____ No
3. Are there gloves for universal precautions in every exam room?
   a. _____ Yes b. _____ No

sues may be highlighted. Then, the specific questions guided by the standards of professional organizations and the litigation history should be explored. Finally, the department's occurrence record and claims history should be evaluated to determine unique problem areas within the institution. Again, this system allows the risk manager to combine the structure, process, and outcome approaches to measuring quality. This systems-oriented approach broadens the scope of analysis and lends credibility to the results.

This section depicts critical elements for review of several conventional areas of risk within a hospital. For each high-risk specialty discussed, specific elements to be included in the departmental review are identified. Then, a list of specific occurrences is given as an example of what types of data could be tracked from incident reports and medical record screens.

Anesthesiology

In the practice of anesthesiology, physicians and certified registered nurse anesthetists administer potent muscle relaxants, sedatives, and anesthetizing agents so that surgical and other invasive procedures may be performed. The inherent risks of this specialty include incorrect administration of agents; inadequate monitoring of the patient, resulting in long-term neurologic sequelae; tooth damage; corneal damage; nerve or muscle injuries; untoward reactions to anesthetics or other medications; and problems associated with equipment malfunction.

In order to promote patient safety, the American Society of Anesthesiologists has promulgated standards related to the type of anesthesia delivery system used and the monitoring of patients required.[2] In addition, the Food and Drug Administration has issued recommendations for checking equipment prior to each case.[3] As a result of these national efforts,

Exhibit 5-5 In-Patient Risk Assessment Survey—Unit Inspection Form

---

UNIT INSPECTION FORM

Person completing form: _____ Date: _____

Location: _____

General:
1. Can conversations among health care personnel or between health care personnel and patients be overheard from patients' rooms?
   a. _____ Yes   b. _____ No
2. Are the halls and patients' rooms quiet and free of boisterous behavior?
   a. _____ Yes   b. _____ No
3. Is there a treatment room for invasive procedures on the unit?
   a. _____ Yes   b. _____ No
4. Do all hospital employees wear name tags?
   a. _____ Yes   b. _____ No
5. Are there exam gloves for universal precautions in every patient room?
   a. _____ Yes   b. _____ No

Readiness for emergencies:
1. Is the emergency cart centrally located on the unit?
   a. _____ Yes   b. _____ No
2. Are intubation trays equipped with
   a. a laryngoscope and extra batteries?   _____ Yes _____ No
   b. appropriately sized endotracheal tubes and scope sights (i.e., adult or pediatric)?   _____ Yes _____ No
3. Is the emergency cart locked?
   a. _____ Yes   b. _____ No
4. Is there a list on top of the cart indicating when the entire cart was last checked?
   a. _____ Yes   b. _____ No
5. Does the unit have the following emergency equipment in a centrally located area:
   a. Emergency O_2 flow meter and tubing   _____ Yes _____ No
      (Where medical gases are available. If no gases, look for O_2 tank.)
   b. Face masks   _____ Yes _____ No
   c. Electrocardiograph (EKG)   _____ Yes _____ No
   d. Defibrillator   _____ Yes _____ No

Medication control:
1. Are prescription pads kept out of sight of patients?
   a. _____ Yes   b. _____ No
2. Are syringes kept out of sight of patients?
   a. _____ Yes   b. _____ No
3. Is there a locked medication room or cart?
   a. _____ Yes   b. _____ No
4. Is there a locked narcotics cabinet on the unit?
   a. _____ Yes   b. _____ No
5. Is there an up-to-date narcotics record used for signing out controlled substances?
   a. _____ Yes   b. _____ No
6. Are the narcotics counted by an RN and another nurse at the end of each shift?
   a. _____ Yes   b. _____ No
7. Are antibiotics and opened vials of medications stored in the refrigerator, if required?
   a. _____ Yes   b. _____ No

Exhibit 5-5 continued

8. Are there sealed receptacles for disposal of syringes and needles in the medication room, on the cart, and in utility rooms?
   a. _____ Yes   b. _____ No
9. Are there special waste containers in the medication room for disposal of chemo-therapeutic agents and contaminated syringes and tubing?
   a. _____ Yes   b. _____ No

COMMENTS:

questions that should be added to the general risk assessment survey include these:[4]

- Are preanesthesia and postanesthesia assessments made before the time of induction and after the patient's discharge from the recovery area?
- Are measurements of a patient's oxygen saturation, blood pressure (noninvasive), heart rate, and temperature obtained and documented during the anesthetic period?
- Are preanesthesia equipment checks performed and documented to evaluate the operational safety of the equipment?
- Are positioning protocols used to prevent nerve and muscle injuries?
- Is a gas analyzer used on every anesthesia delivery system?
- Are gas scavenging systems used to prevent the leaching of nitrous oxide into the operating room environment?
- Are preventive maintenance logs kept for all anesthesia equipment?
- Are disconnect and parameter alarms used for all patients undergoing general anesthesia?

In addition, adverse patient outcomes potentially or actually related to inadequate monitoring or equipment failure should be reviewed in the quality assurance process of the department. Some clinical indicators and incidents that could be monitored and reviewed in departmental quality assurance/risk management meetings include[5]

- difficult intubation or intubation-related mechanical trauma
- reintubation

Exhibit 5-6 Ambulatory Care Risk Assessment Survey—Clinic Nursing
Supervisor Interview

CLINIC NURSING SUPERVISOR INTERVIEW

Person conducting interview: _____ Date: _____
Clinic Supervisor: _____ Location: _____

Appointments:
1. Is there an established written procedure for follow-up of missed or broken
   appointments?
   a. _____ Yes   b. _____ No
   IF YES, PLEASE DESCRIBE: _____

   _____

   _____.

2. When there is follow-up with patients for missed appointments, is the response
   recorded in the chart?
   a. _____ Yes   b. _____ No
   IF YES, PLEASE DESCRIBE FORMAT: _____

   _____

   _____.

3. Is there a patient reminder system for yearly (or scheduled) examinations?
   a. _____ Yes   b. _____ No
   IF YES, PLEASE DESCRIBE SYSTEM: _____

   _____

   _____.

4. Are new patients scheduled within two weeks of the request for an appointment?
   a. _____ Yes   b. _____ No
5. Are new patients given information about clinic check-in procedures?
   a. _____ Yes   b. _____ No
6. Is there a system for follow-up on clinical lab or test results?
   a. _____ Yes   b. _____ No
   TYPES OF RESULTS AND METHOD FOR FOLLOW-UP: _____

   _____

   _____

Charts:
1. Is there a work area or station where notes or dictation may be made without the
   potential of patients seeing or overhearing confidential information?
   a. _____ Yes   b. _____ No
2. Do the clerical staff personnel file clinic notes in the charts before returning the
   charts to the Medical Records Department?
   a. _____ Yes   b. _____ No
3. Are telephone contacts recorded in the patients' charts?
   a. _____ Yes   b. _____ No

Exhibit 5-6 continued

Medication control:
1. Is there a written policy for disposal of chemotherapeutic agents, as well as contaminated IV bags and tubing syringes?
   a. _____ Yes   b. _____ No
   IF YES, PLEASE DESCRIBE: _____

_____.

Emergencies:
1. Are all staff members up to date via yearly retraining sessions for CPR?
   a. _____ Yes   b. _____ No
   IF NO, EXPLAIN: _____

_____

COMMENTS:

- aspiration
- dental injuries
- ocular injuries
- nerve or muscle damage
- wide swings in hemodynamic and respiratory parameters
- cardiac arrest in the operating or recovery room
- equipment malfunction during case
- unplanned admission to the intensive care unit
- transfusion reaction
- medication error or adverse reaction

Obstetrics

Another specialty area with known risk exposure is the area of obstetrics. Most of the allegations encountered in lawsuits deal with the failure to properly monitor an infant during the labor process, the failure to diagnose and treat problems of pregnancy, and the delay or failure to perform a Caesarean section delivery.[6] Because this has become a highly litigious area, the American College of Obstetricians and Gynecologists has set forth standards for perinatal care.[7] In order to determine a hospital's level of risk exposure with respect to these national standards, the following questions should be explored during a departmental risk assessment review:

- Do all patients who present to the obstetrics or emergency department later than 20 weeks' gestation receive a baseline electronic fetal monitor (EFM) assessment?
- Are all high-risk patients monitored continuously with EFM?
- Does the hospital-based clinic have a protocol for screening high-risk patients?
- Are physicians and nurses who are responsible for interpreting fetal monitoring strips trained for such interpretation?
- Is an anesthesiologist available at all times for emergency Caesarean section deliveries?
- Can a Caesarean section delivery be performed within 30 minutes at any time?
- Are there policies governing the administration of oxytocic agents?
- Is there an active in-service program on infant resuscitation for all delivery room personnel? Is infant resuscitation equipment available in all delivery rooms?

In addition, it is important to institute a process of ongoing monitoring of quality through the review of specific cases. (This process should include practitioners in obstetrics, pediatrics or neonatology, and anesthesia.) Types of occurrences that could be tracked for quality assurance purposes include[8]

- Apgar scores of 3 or less at five minutes
- eclampsia
- maternal lacerations greater than second degree
- other maternal injuries or complications
- infant injuries during delivery
- maternal or fetal death
- oxytocin use without concomitant monitoring
- lack of a baseline EFM assessment
- babies delivered at less than 34 weeks' gestation
- second stage of labor longer than 2.5 hours

Psychiatry

The psychiatric specialty has become an area of high risk for professional liability litigation. With the multitude of settings and treatment modalities for psychiatric treatment, there is extreme variability in the types of allegations made against psychiatrists and other mental health workers. Some of these include the failure to provide proper follow-up after discharge from an in-patient setting, improper treatment with pharmacologic agents, premature release from psychiatric care, failure to adequately supervise suicidal or destructive patients, failure to warn others of violent behaviors, and the improper or inappropriate use of electroconvulsive therapy.[9] In addition, recent cases suggest a rise of claims alleging inappropriate sexual behavior both of patients and of staff.

Given this array of potential allegations, the following questions should be added to the departmental survey:

- Does the hospital have specific policies and procedures for the involuntary commitment of patients?
- Are there specific policies and procedures for the protection of confidential patient information?
- Are there specific procedures for the institution of suicide precautions and various types of patient observation?
- Are seclusion and restraint policies routinely reviewed and evaluated?
- Are windows in the units securely fastened and tamper proof?
- Are sharp objects (i.e., needles, scissors, knives, OT/PT equipment) routinely counted on all psychiatric units?
- Is there a procedure for referring patients to out-patient psychiatric providers?
- Is there an active in-service program for training personnel in how to react in a crisis situation?
- Is written consent required for each series of electroconvulsive therapy?
- Is there a clear policy for the reporting of adverse effects from psychopharmacologic agents?
- Are blood levels of potentially toxic drugs measured routinely?

In addition to verifying that the appropriate policies and procedures exist to protect patients from injury, the department of psychiatry should routinely evaluate adverse outcomes to determine if actions should be taken to alter or enhance current practices. Clinical indicators that could be used to identify potential quality of care problems include[10]

- death of a psychiatric in-patient
- cardiac or respiratory arrest of an in-patient
- attempted or successful suicide attempt while on the unit
- elopement from the unit or failure to return from authorized outings
- inappropriate sexual conduct of in-patients
- adverse reactions or sequelae from psychopharmacologic agents
- incorrect procedure followed during involuntary commitment
- unexpected transfer to a medical unit for a previously undiagnosed medical problem
- violent acts against self or others after discharge from psychiatric care

Ambulatory Care Facilities

With the increase in emphasis on out-patient procedures and evaluations, there has been a parallel rise in the number of hospital-sponsored ambulatory care facilities. This shift from traditional in-patient care to treatment in out-patient settings relates to many factors, including the change of reimbursement methods and the spread of health maintenance organizations. As the number of out-patient visits increases, there is a need to control the risks associated with the episodic and patient-driven nature of such encounters. Because of the high volume of patients in out-patient settings, there may be delays in a patient's obtaining an appointment or instances in which inadequate examinations are performed. Further, the lack of continuity of care in such settings may hinder the ability of the provider to make accurate and complete assessment of the patient's condition.[11]

The risks associated with ambulatory care include the potential for delays or omissions in diagnosis and treatment, for miscommunication with the patient leading to adverse outcomes, and for complications of treatment.[12] To evaluate these risks, several questions should be added to the interview list for ambulatory care areas. Many of these are reflected in the general risk assessment tools for ambulatory care, particularly in the Clinic Nursing Supervisor Interview guide (Exhibit 5-6). In addition, the following items are relevant:

- Is there a method for documenting the advice given during telephone conversations with patients?

- Are the manufacturer and lot number of a vaccination serum documented according to the rules of the National Childhood Vaccine Injury Act?
- Are learners such as residents and medical students supervised by faculty members or attending physicians in the clinic?
- Are the problem lists at the front of patients' charts kept current?
- Is emergency equipment well maintained, and do staff attend regular in-service education programs to ensure quick response in the event of a cardiac arrest or other life-threatening event?
- Is there a system for timely review of radiology, pathology, or laboratory results by the responsible physician or physician extender?
- Is informed consent obtained for all invasive procedures performed in the ambulatory care setting?
- Is there a written policy for dealing with prescription refills?

Departments must establish means to review occurrences in the out-patient setting as well as those in the hospital in-patient areas. Some of the occurrence screens that could be used include[13]

- all deaths, as well as all cardiac or respiratory arrests in the ambulatory care area
- unexpected admission or emergency room visit following an out-patient visit
- patient falls
- medication or transfusion errors or adverse reactions
- adverse outcomes related to procedures/surgery
- lack of written consent for invasive procedures
- intravenous fluid infiltration resulting in tissue damage

Emergency Departments

In emergency departments (EDs) at community hospitals, as well as at trauma centers, the issues outlined for ambulatory care facilities must be supplemented with attention to risks associated with the often critical condition of acutely ill patients who present for emergent, lifesaving care. Decisions related to such care must often be made rapidly in the context of crisis situations (and often with little, if any, knowledge of a patient's preexisting problems). This high-intensity atmosphere means added risk exposure for the practitioners in such settings. Allegations against emergency department physicians frequently focus on the failure to diagnose such life-threatening or potentially critical conditions as spinal fractures, foreign bodies, infections (e.g., meningitis, sepsis, pneumonia), appendicitis, ectopic pregnancies, and myocardial infarction.[14] Other allegations may relate to decisions made regarding discharge from or treatments rendered in the ED setting.

Questions directed toward the medical director and the nursing supervisor of the ED during a risk assessment evaluation should include these:

- Are policies and procedures in place to govern the triage process and the monitoring of patients?
- Are all patients who present to the ED triaged, and is there a medical record generated for each?
- Is there a method for ensuring that the results of laboratory tests and radiology studies are documented in the medical record, along with a physician's interpretation of the findings?
- Is a physician involved in the care of all patients who are seen in the ED?
- Are all staff required to be certified in the Advanced Cardiac Life Support?
- Are follow-up visits scheduled in the ED or in associated clinics? If patients are seen in other areas after the ED visit, how are the medical records transferred?
- Is there a system for follow-up with patients if initial findings or diagnoses differ from the final reports?
- Are discharge instructions to the patient clearly documented in the ED record?
- If the hospital is a trauma center, are there policies and procedures governing the communication among specialty disciplines? Is there a quick-response trauma team available 24 hours a day? Are all patient care reviews of trauma patients performed by all specialties involved?
- If the ED supports an air transport program, are the policies and procedures related to communication, transport, and safety routinely reviewed and evaluated? Is a flight team consisting of qualified, trained personnel available at all hours?

The types of ED occurrences that should be monitored in an ongoing quality assurance and loss prevention program are as follows:[15]

- all deaths in the ED
- unscheduled return to the ED within 24 hours for the same or similar complaint

- death within 48 hours following discharge from the ED
- delay or error in diagnosis related to misinterpretation of radiographs, lab results, or electrocardiograms
- patient leaving the ED against medical advice
- patient falling in the ED
- patient presenting with complaint or history of head trauma discharged in an altered state of consciousness
- lack of proper consent for invasive procedure
- untoward results from treatment in the ED

Hospital-Sponsored Home Health Care

The provision of home health care is an emerging area of liability exposure that should be considered by risk managers in institutions that sponsor this type of service. With the national trend toward earlier discharge of patients under the Medicare-approved prospective payment system, the number of home health programs has increased dramatically since 1983. Accompanying this shift toward provision of care in the home are several risks associated with treatments given in the absence of constant, direct supervision. As such, the following items should be included in a risk assessment of any hospital-sponsored home care program:[16]

- Are there specific protocols for admitting patients to a home care program?
- Are treatment plans specifically outlined and approved by a supervising physician?
- Is there complete documentation of care, with summaries sent to the treating physician?
- Are there policies and procedures governing the discharge of patients from the care of the agency?
- Is there an inspection and preventive maintenance program for all equipment used by patients in the home environment?
- Are personnel and family members trained in handling emergency situations?

In addition to these survey questions, a quality assurance program should be designed to review unexpected occurrences in the home. Some of the indicators serving to prompt review include[17]

- unexpected death of a patient while receiving home care
- injury to the patient due to improper use of equipment

- unexpected admission to the hospital due to a worsening condition
- medication error or reaction
- recurrent or worsening infection
- delayed healing or dehiscence of a surgical wound
- patient or family complaints regarding providers

CONCLUSION

This chapter has outlined a process for evaluating the risk potential of specific departments associated with a hospital. Each individual area has unique risk exposures that require attention by the risk manager. In addition, a risk manager must be prepared to evaluate the possible risks associated with new technologies acquired by and new business ventures undertaken by the institution.

J.E. Orlikoff and A.M. Vanagunas outline criteria for identifying future areas of risk exposure.[18] These criteria identify services for which demand is increasing dramatically, for which there is a potential for serious injury to the patient, or for which there are undeveloped or underdeveloped standards of care. Once high-risk areas are identified, a hospital risk management program can assist in developing systems, protocols, and procedures to prevent liability. It is imperative that risk managers monitor the changing scene of health care in order to be prepared for and prevent losses and patient injury. This type of proactive approach can be linked with quality improvement efforts to head off catastrophic incidents.

NOTES

1. Health Care Financing Administration, *Quality Screens* (Washington, D.C.: Government Printing Office, 1986).

2. Joyce Riffer, "Anesthesia Monitoring Standards: A Quality Issue," *Hospitals* (Nov. 5, 1986): 76.

3. Food and Drug Administration, *Anesthesia Apparatus Checkout Recommendations* (1986).

4. B. Youngberg, *Preacquisition Questions,* Dec. 1987 (photocopy).

5. L. Sabnis and J.A. Aldrete, "Letter to the Editor," *APSF Newsletter* (June 1988): 10; B. Youngberg, "Anesthesia Monthly Quality Monitors," Dec. 1987 (photocopy); Joint Commission on Accreditation of Healthcare Organizations, "Task Force Sights New Quality Horizons," *Agenda for Change Update* 2, no. 1.

6. J. Goldberg, and G.P. Kraus, "Developing and Implementing a Comprehensive Risk Prevention Program," in *Health Care Risk Management: Organization and Claims Administration,* G.P. Kraus, ed. (Md.: Rynd Communications, 1986).

7. American College of Obstetricians and Gynecologists, *Standards for Obstetric Gynecologic Services.* 6th ed. (Washington, D.C.: American College of Obstetricians and Gynecologists, 1985).

8. B. Youngberg, "Maternal-Fetal Monthly Quality Monitors," Dec. 1987 (photocopy).

9. S. Lieberman, "Psychiatric Risk Control," in *The Pulse: Topics in Healthcare Risk Management,* vol. 3, no. 2 (Dallas, Tex.: Alexander and Alexander, Inc., 1988).

10. B. Youngberg, "Psychiatric Quality Monitors," Dec. 1987 (photocopy).

11. W.F. Jessee, "Quality Assurance/Risk Management: Interactions in Ambulatory Care Settings" (Paper delivered at the National Conference on Quality Assurance in Ambulatory Health Care: Joint Commission on Accreditation of Healthcare Organizations, Nov. 9–10, 1987).

12. S.L. Read-Triebsch, "Risk Exposure in Ambulatory Care," *Perspectives in Healthcare Risk Management* (Fall 1987): 5.

13. "Guidelines for Outpatient Reportable Occurrences," University of Colorado Health Sciences Center, March 1988 (photocopy).

14. J.D. Dunn, "Risk Management in Emergency Medicine," *Emergency Medicine Clinics of North America* 5, no. 1 (Feb. 1987): 51–69.

15. B. Youngberg, "Emergency Department Quality Monitors," Dec. 1987 (photocopy). "Guidelines for Emergency Room Reportable Occurrences," University of Colorado Health Sciences Center, Nov. 1988 (photocopy).

16. American Hospital Association, "Managing Risks and Quality in Hospital-Sponsored Home Care " (Chicago: American Hospital Association, 1987).

17. B. Youngberg, "Home Care Quality Monitors," June 1988 (photocopy).

18. J.E. Orlikoff, and A.M. Vanagunas, "Predicting the Future of Hospital Liability," *Trustee* (Sept. 1988): 8–19.

PART III

Developing Tools To Manage Risk

Part III begins with a chapter delineating the steps taken by the University of Wisconsin Hospital and Clinics in Madison, Wisconsin, to implement a model program for integrating the disciplines of quality assurance and risk management. It describes all of the elements of program design and implementation, including the approaches that worked best and those that were problematic. The final result of the program and the "Occurrence Screen" it produced (included in this chapter) should provide the reader with an excellent process to use to establish a similar program. The policy and procedure for the screen's implementation are also included.

The two succeeding chapters discuss the importance of education both for staff and the consumer and describe the process for setting up educational programs that will provide additional support for the risk management effort. Clearly, well-defined and well-implemented educational plans will contribute significantly to the success of the hospital's loss control and quality of care programs.

chapter 6

Development of an Occurrence Screen Tool To Integrate Quality Assurance and Risk Management

Ann R. Mansfield
Ann L. Schoofs

THE RATIONALE FOR DEVELOPING A MODEL PROGRAM

Risk management in health care has undergone an extensive evolution. In a short period of time the emphasis in risk management has changed dramatically from a reactive to a proactive focus, and its scope has been expanded beyond claims investigation to claims prevention. Usually one person (who often had many additional responsibilities) was designated to respond to situations where an adverse outcome could result in potential liability. For example, any situation where a patient was injured in the course of treatment could trigger investigations by risk management. Then, to facilitate documentation and early warning of patient injuries, adverse outcomes, or unexpected occurrences, incident reporting was developed. The incidents reported, however, were usually medication errors; falls and slips; and incorrect sponge, needle, or instrument counts. Unfortunately these data correlated little with claims actually filed or dollars paid out by the hospital for claims. Furthermore, the information was rarely compiled in a manner sufficient to identify problems, trigger appropriate follow-up, or prevent claims.

Recently, the value of developing a system for claims and/or risk prevention has been recognized in health care. Many health care providers are facing the challenge of developing an effective risk management mechanism to achieve this outcome.

At the same time that risk management was evolving, quality assurance was gaining greater attention because of extensive changes occurring in the health care regulatory environment. Rapid advances in health care technology, the growth of medical specialties in the health care environment, and the dramatic rise in malpractice litigation contributed to the need for more structured internal peer review activities.[1] In 1979 the Joint Commission on Accreditation of Hospitals (Joint Commission) added a quality assurance standard that outlined a problem-focused approach. Over time the standard has evolved from one discouraging integration of risk management and quality assurance information within an institution to one requiring their integration. As Dr. William Jessee of the Joint Commission has aptly commented, "Linking Quality Assurance with Risk Management is like improving the weather: Everyone agrees it's a good idea, but hardly anyone seems to know how to go about it."[2]

The method of integrating risk management with quality assurance varies by institution. For example, in some settings one person has responsibility for both areas, in other situations the two roles rarely interact, and in yet other organizations, risk management and quality assurance function independently but work cooperatively. In most situations, regardless of the organizational structure, the two areas collect and have interest in similar information. It is this overlap that led to the logical development of the "Occurrence Screen" (a tool to identify adverse hospital incidents) at the University of Wisconsin Hospital and Clinics. (See Appendix 6-A.) An explanation of the development process and its philosophy follows.

INTRODUCTION

Since the early 1970s the concept of integrating quality assurance and risk management has been discussed in the literature. The literature supports the fact that the increase in litigation for bad outcomes regardless of the presence of negligence lends itself well to peer review activities. It is also known that these activities (1) contribute to identifying problems that pose quality of care and other potential litigation concerns and (2) assist in future quality assurance program development. This exchange creates an opportunity for developing predictive and preventive indicators in risk management and for optimizing quality assurance efforts. Ultimately, risk to patients and providers is minimized, and the delivery of quality is assured.[3] Because of the emphasis on quality assurance, recognition of the quality information offered by risk management, and Joint Commission requirements, it is now appropriate and indeed necessary to develop a system to integrate risk management and quality assurance.[4]

The purpose of this chapter is to describe the mechanism developed at the University of Wisconsin Hospital and Clinics (UWHC) to achieve what UWHC believes is an excellent cornerstone for the integration of quality assurance and risk management. Although this system may not work for everyone, we believe that, with adaptations, it could work for most. We do know that it requires at the very least a close working relationship between the departments of quality assurance and risk management.

RISK MANAGEMENT AND QUALITY ASSURANCE AT THE UNIVERSITY OF WISCONSIN HOSPITAL AND CLINICS

The University of Wisconsin Hospital and Clinics is a 503-bed facility located in Madison. Annually there are approximately 16,000 admissions and 350,000 clinic visits. Although the director of Quality Assurance and the director of Risk Management report to different hospital administrators, there is a strong informal link and a spirit of cooperation between the two departments. In addition, while the University Legal Services Department is not directly involved in daily hospital risk management activities, it functions in an advisory capacity to the Risk Management Department.

The Risk Management Department is responsible for all aspects of claims management and prevention, including investigation of the following areas: professional liability, general liability, and workers' compensation. The department consists of the director and an assistant.

The Quality Assurance Department is responsible for providing direct support and staffing to all medical staff peer review activities. Medical Record Department coders and Utilization Review coordinators support the data collection function. Quality Assurance staff provide nonmedical staff departments with education and feedback regarding quality assurance.

For a number of years the sharing of information between Risk Management and Quality Assurance was limited to the Quality Evaluation and Review Committee (the quality assurance committee of the medical staff), which reviewed incident reports on a quarterly basis. In early 1986 the directors of Quality Assurance and Risk Management began meeting monthly to discuss morbidity and mortality data and other quality assurance and risk management information, before and after the clinical departmental peer review process. In these meetings an attempt was also made to utilize incident reporting to verify and/or substantiate quality assurance and utilization review information. For example, significant incidents noted in the medical record were compared retrospectively with incident reports filed.

Regular interaction between the Quality Assurance and Risk Management departments resulted in a close working relationship. Both departments realized the mutual benefit of sharing the above information and began to evaluate other hospital reporting systems. The primary objectives were to assess duplication in reporting and to explore what other information was being collected. The monitoring systems evaluated included incident reports, "less-than-effective service" reports, and various quality assurance monitors. Although it was not a "monitor," informal reporting by telephone or memo to the directors of Risk Management or Quality Assurance was occurring. This was also considered.

Within a short period of time, both departments became frustrated with the existing incident reporting system, for the following reasons:

1. Reporting was not timely.
2. The incident report form was complicated and for that reason was often not completed properly.
3. Incidents seemed essentially restricted to medication errors; falls; and incorrect sponge, needle, or instrument counts.
4. Incident reporting was not serving as an effective early warning system for potential claims. There was no correlation between incidents, quality assurance data, and actual claims.
5. The reporting process was viewed as punitive by the staff.
6. There was limited or no meaningful follow-up to persons and departments involved in reporting incidents.
7. Reporting by physicians was nonexistent.

In addition to the incident report, a less-than-effective service report was utilized to notify other departments of inadequate service. This form provided one-way communication to the "less than effective" department and was often used to direct anger at another department or to focus blame for a mishap. An inherent weakness with this problem identification mechanism was the lack of feedback to the initiator regarding problem resolution. Frequently it failed to result in needed changes in the system, as had been originally intended.

Additionally, after discharge Medical Record Department staff routinely reviewed charts, using quality assurance monitors for cases of documented problems or potential problems in the delivery of care provided (retrospective review). These cases were referred to clinical departmental peer review committees for further review and determination of the quality of care provided. An inherent weakness in this process was the untimeliness of the review.

The directors of Quality Assurance and Risk Management recognized that many of the data collection efforts of their two departments were duplicative. Clearly the two departments were operating independently of each other and not experiencing the mutual benefit of sharing information in a meaningful and complementary manner. These departments were interested not only in collecting more pertinent data but also in decreasing duplicative activities and in changing the philosophy of reporting away from the punitive mindset to something more constructive, by placing greater emphasis on improving the quality of patient care. Therefore, the directors of Quality Assurance and Risk Management proposed that a task force be appointed to address these identified issues.

Task Force

Support from the medical staff and administration was recognized as essential to introducing the concept of quality assurance/risk management integration. Therefore, the directors of Risk Management and Quality Assurance sought support from key persons in the organization: the associate dean/director of Clinical Affairs, the chairperson of the Quality Evaluation and Review Committee, and appropriate hospital administrators. Upon receiving approval from these people, the directors of Quality Assurance and Risk Management were named cochairpersons of the task force. A group was appointed and intentionally limited to a few key people representing the Risk Management and Quality Assurance departments, Pharmacy, and Nursing. Pharmacy and Nursing included the largest group of reporters utilizing incident and less-than-effective service reports, so their involvement was recognized to be crucial. The goal was to meet frequently, work efficiently, and maintain the momentum of the group process. At the same time, meetings were held with key medical staff to inform them of task force progress and recent Quality Assurance and Risk Management activities and to gain their support and input.

The task force gave attention to issues identified by the directors of Risk Management and Quality Assurance, focusing on the development of a tool that would replace incident reporting, less-than-effective service reporting, and quality assurance monitoring. Incorporated into this objective was the goal of effecting change in the philosophy of reporting. In addition, another goal was to combine three existing systems into a single reporting mechanism. It then became logical for the task force to develop a tool and an accompanying system that would meet the above-stated objectives and serve to integrate quality assurance and risk management reporting at UWHC.

The first objective of the task force was to educate Nursing and Pharmacy task force members about the proposed concept of "integration" and the objectives of the project. In preparing for this, a review of the literature was conducted. Additionally, incident reports and quality assurance monitoring information from comparable hospitals were obtained and reviewed.

The concept of integration met with some resistance and skepticism within the committee. This primarily related to the reporting of incidents or situations that were not traditionally reported by hospital staff (nonphysicians). For example, one task force member expressed great concern regarding nonphysicians using a form that could be used to report unexpected deaths, surgical or procedure outcomes, cardiac or respiratory arrests, and the like. This concern was resolved when task force members understood that physicians would review these and other clinically related situations prior to a report being submitted. After approximately four months, it was felt that all members of the task force fully understood and advocated the concepts of integration.

The early work of the task force also focused on the need for hospital-wide education to achieve an understanding of the proposed integration. Special attention was given to soliciting feedback from medical staff, various peer review committees, administration, and department representatives. Task force members identified and met with key individuals in the organization to introduce an initial draft of the data collection tool and to discuss its use. The goal was to obtain feedback from virtually every department.

Throughout the development of the data collection tool, the task force constantly referred to the following objectives:

1. Design a form (data collection tool), keeping it and the entire reporting phase as simple as possible. (It was believed that this would enhance complete reporting, compared to the previous experience with more complicated incident reports.)
2. Incorporate information from four previously existing mechanisms:
   • incident reports
   • quality assurance monitors
   • less-than-effective service reports
   • informal reporting (telephone calls or memos to Risk Management and Quality Assurance)
3. Streamline the documentation of risk management and quality assurance information and incorporate three forms into one

4. Provide a simple mechanism for communicating interdepartmentally at the time of an occurrence or incident
5. Provide a process for case finding and peer review
6. Enhance the effectiveness of reporting to achieve the following:
   - timely reporting and feedback
   - valid, high-quality information
   - improved interdepartmental information
   - a centralized computer database for generating reports
7. Decrease the frustration of collecting and reporting of meaningless data (i.e., information that does not correlate with quality of care issues and/or claims)

Occurrence Screen System

An occurrence screen system was developed and implemented to formalize the integration of Risk Management and Quality Assurance by mid-1988. It consisted of a reporting or data collection tool—the Occurrence Screen—and a specially designed computer program utilizing dBase III-Plus for report generation. The name "Occurrence Screen" was chosen to distinguish the new concept from the traditional incident report. It was also believed that the name would have a less negative connotation.

The Occurrence Screen is a single-sided form with two carbonless copies. The copies are immediately sent to individual department(s) involved in an occurrence to communicate the occurrence and enhance timely follow-up. On the back of the form are definitions of potentially misleading or unclear occurrences (e.g., "unexpected neuro deficit not present upon admission: instance when a patient is discharged with a neurological deficit that was not present on admission and is not considered a normal consequence of the prescribed medical/surgical intervention"). In addition, there are directions on form completion, use, and routing. (See Exhibits 6-1 and 6-2.)

The Occurrence Screen underwent numerous revisions before its final form was set, as a result of meeting with and obtaining feedback from key members of the medical staff and representatives from nearly every hospital department. By the time the Occurrence Screen and a proposal to pilot it were presented to the Medical Board's Quality Evaluation and Review Committee, nearly every department head and numerous medical staff members had provided input into its use and design. It is believed that because of this process, the Quality Evaluation and Review Committee was supportive and approved the Occurrence Screen for a pilot study. In addition to the Quality Evaluation and Review Committee's approval, it

Exhibit 6-1 University of Wisconsin Hospital and Clinics Occurrence Screen

---

I. PATIENT
INFORMATION

Inpatient-Service: _____   Attending Physician: _____
Outpatient-Clinic: _____   Physician Contacted: _____
Visitor: _____   Person(s) Involved: _____
Other: _____   Department(s) Involved:
_____

Date/Time of Occurrence: _____   Location: _____
Patient's Level of Consciousness: _____   Restraints/Siderails Used (Explain): ___

---

* = THESE OCCURRENCES REQUIRE PHYSICIAN REVIEW
AND STATEMENT

II. TYPE OF OCCURRENCE:
- ☐ *Unexpected Cardiac/Respiratory Arrest
- ☐ *Unexpected Death
- ☐ *Unexpected Hemorrhage (Requiring Transfusion)
- ☐ *Unexpected Surgical/Procedure Outcome
- ☐ *Unexpected Anesthetic Outcome
- ☐ *Unexpected Atelectasis/ Pneumothorax/Aspiration (Requiring Treatment)
- ☐ *Unexpected Neuro Deficit Not Present on Admission
- ☐ *Unexpected Blood Transfusion Reaction
- ☐ *Reaction to Contrast/Dye Type: _____
- ☐ *Wound Dehiscence
- ☐ *Nonscheduled Return to OR/ Hospital/Clinic/ER
- ☐ *Deep Vein Thrombosis/Phlebitis
- ☐ *Skin Breakdown
- ☐ *Incorrect Blood Administration
- ☐ *Incorrect Sponge/Needle Count
- ☐ *Slip and/or Fall
- ☐ *Injury to Patient/Visitor
- ☐ *Other—Specify: _____
- ☐ Incomplete/Incorrect/Missing Consent
- ☐ Left Without Service/Elopement/ AMA
- ☐ Problems Related to Inter-unit Patient Transfer (Explain in Narrative)
- ☐ Equipment/Supply: Malfunction/ Inadequate Stock

- ☐ Delay in/Inadequate: Service/ Consult
- ☐ Irate Patient/Family/Friends
- ☐ Personal Property Loss/Damage
- ☐ Other—Specify: _____

DIAGNOSTIC/THERAPEUTIC SERVICES:
SERVICE: _____
- ☐ *Incorrect Procedure/Test/ Therapy
- ☐ *Incorrect Test Result/Reading
- ☐ *Incorrect Diagnosis Made
- ☐ Sample Contamination
- ☐ Other—Specify: _____

MEDICATIONS/I.V. SOLUTIONS:
TYPE OF OCCURRENCE:
- ☐ *Adverse Drug Experience
- ☐ *Incorrect Patient
- ☐ *Incorrect Drug/Solution
- ☐ *Incorrect Dosage/Rate
- ☐ *Incorrect Time
- ☐ *Incorrect Route
- ☐ *Omission
- ☐ *Drug Extravasation
- ☐ *Other—Specify: _____

REASON GIVEN FOR DRUG OCCURRENCE:
- ☐ Did Not Read Profile/Label
- ☐ Transcription Error
- ☐ Dispensing Error
- ☐ Incorrect Administration
- ☐ Other—Specify: _____

Exhibit 6-1 continued

III. BRIEF NARRATIVE: (Statement of Facts Only—Additional Space on Reverse Side)

SIGNATURE/DATE:

IV. *PHYSICIAN/OTHER PROVIDER STATEMENT OF OCCURRENCE: (Check Appropriate One(s)—Explain in Narrative)
_____ NO INJURY _____ FIRST AID _____ DIAGNOSTIC TEST(S) _____ TREATMENT REQUIRED

SIGNATURE/DATE:

V. FOLLOW-UP TO PATIENT/VISITOR/OTHER: (Additional Space on Reverse Side)

SIGNATURE/TITLE:

REVIEWED BY: _____ **DEPARTMENT/TITLE:** _____
DATE: _____
REVIEWED BY: _____ **DEPARTMENT/TITLE:** _____
DATE: _____

ROUTING PROCESS: WHITE COPY—SEND TO F6/258 (TUBE #68) WITHIN 24 HOURS
COPIES SENT TO DEPARTMENTS: _____ *(YELLOW)* _____ *(PINK)*

Source: Courtesy of University of Wisconsin Hospital and Clinics, Madison, Wisconsin.

---

was felt that the entire medical staff needed to be informed and prepared for the pilot study. The Occurrence Screen was presented to and reviewed with the chairperson of every clinical department and nearly every medical staff committee as well. Some of the initial feedback was skeptical. Several physicians were concerned about nonphysicians reporting clinically related information, such as nurses reporting an "unexpected surgical/procedure outcome." They were also concerned about providing adequate definitions for some of the occurrences, such as "unexpected hemorrhage," "unexplained anesthetic outcome," and the like. It was emphasized by the directors of Quality Assurance and Risk Management that there was no intention of promoting an adversarial relationship between physicians and nonphysicians. For the "medical occurrences" (as noted with an asterisk on the form), a physician would be required to review the Occurrence Screen prior to its being submitted to the Quality Assurance and Risk Management departments.

Exhibit 6-2 Directions for Use of Occurrence Screen

DIRECTIONS: Please complete the first three sections of this form before promptly providing it to your supervisor or the person designated for further review. The back side of this form can be used any time additional space is necessary. A separate form should be completed for each occurrence.

SECTION I:
- Address-o-graph plate can be used for in/out patients.
- The attending staff physician's name is requested.
- "Level of consciousness" choices: agitated, confused, depressed, mentally impaired, oriented, sedated, unconscious, other.

SECTION II: Mark all appropriate occurrences. When a category has more than one option, i.e., "unexpected cardiac/respiratory arrest," circle the appropriate choice(s) to identify the specific occurrence.
* = Occurrence requires physician review and statement.

SECTION III: Completed by person initiating the form.

SECTION IV: Completed by physician/other provider (when occurrence in section II is notated with an *) or the supervisor/designated person performing further review if physician statement is not required.

SECTION V: Completed by the person performing subsequent follow-up, per department policy (i.e., for Nursing—Nursing Supervisor I).
ORIGINAL PART OF FORM: Routed to QA/Risk Management (room F6/258—Tube #68) immediately upon completion of Section V.
COPIES 2/3 OF FORM: Concomitantly routed to the appropriate person(s)/department(s) for follow-up and routed to QA/Risk Management (F6/258—Tube #68) upon completion.

"TYPE OF OCCURRENCE" DEFINITIONS:
UNEXPECTED CARDIAC/RESPIRATORY ARREST—Patient, not presently treated in an ICU, who is neither a DO NOT RESUSCITATE nor at known risk for cardiac/respiratory arrest.
UNEXPECTED DEATH—Death occurring in a patient at little/no risk based on prognosis after an initial admission evaluation and work-up.
UNEXPECTED HEMORRHAGE (REQUIRING TRANSFUSION)—An instance in which, although blood loss is recognized as a risk of a procedure or medical intervention, excessive bleeding occurs, requiring a transfusion and/or return to the OR.
UNEXPECTED SURGICAL/PROCEDURE OUTCOME—Outcome of surgery or a procedure was not expected.
UNEXPECTED ANESTHETIC OUTCOME—Outcome of anesthesia was not expected.
UNEXPECTED ATELECTASIS/PNEUMOTHORAX/ASPIRATION (REQUIRING TREATMENT)—Instances in which atelectasis, pneumothorax, or aspiration occurred when it was not considered to be a risk of a medical/surgical intervention, or if a chest tube is placed or patient receives empirical treatment.
UNEXPECTED NEURO DEFICIT NOT PRESENT ON ADMISSION—Instance when a patient is discharged with a neurologic deficit that was not present on admission and is not considered an expected consequence of the prescribed medical/surgical intervention.

Exhibit 6-2 continued

UNEXPECTED BLOOD TRANSFUSION REACTION—Life-threatening or potentially life-threatening (in future treatment) response to a blood transfusion.
REACTION TO CONTRAST/DYE—Life-threatening or potentially life-threatening
(in future treatment) response to a contrast medium/dye used for diagnostic purposes.
WOUND DEHISCENCE—Separation of the layers of a surgical wound, requiring
re-operation/repair.
NONSCHEDULED RETURN TO OR/HOSPITAL/CLINIC/ER—Patient present-
ing emergently to the OR, Hospital, Clinic, or ER, requiring further unexpected
treatment related to a previous visit at UWHC.
DEEP VEIN THROMBOSIS/PHLEBITIS—Not identified on admission, verified
per physician evaluation and/or doppler, requiring treatment such as anticoagulants.
SKIN BREAKDOWN—Skin degeneration that arises during hospitalization, requiring wound packing, dressing changes, surgical intervention, or antibiotic management.
LEFT WITHOUT SERVICE/ELOPEMENT/AMA—Left without service = Patient
electively choosing to leave prior to assessment and/or initiation of treatment.
PROBLEMS RELATED TO INTER-UNIT PATIENT TRANSFER—This may include early discharge from ICU, miscommunication, inadequate communication, etc.
EQUIPMENT/SUPPLY MALFUNCTION/INADEQUATE STOCK—Situation
that adversely affects/delays patient care.
INJURY TO PATIENT/VISITOR—Includes but not limited to suicide attempt, self-
inflicted injury, or mishap resulting in injury to someone other than employee.
INCOMPLETE/INCORRECT/MISSING CONSENT—Required consent in non-
emergent situations.
ADVERSE DRUG EXPERIENCE—Includes both allergic reactions and adverse
drug reactions. For further information see Administrative P&P:8.20.

NARRATIVE/STATEMENT/FOLLOW-UP CONTINUED:

Source: Courtesy of University of Wisconsin Hospital and Clinics, Madison, Wisconsin.

The physicians were also concerned about the implications of reporting
clinical information regarding a physician's practice on a form such as this,
and they questioned whether its confidentiality could be protected. In
response to this concern, the University Legal Services Department was
consulted. It was Legal Services' opinion that the form and system could
be protected as long as a specific policy and procedure approved by the
Medical Board was in place regarding its use and purpose. As further
protection, all reporting information is stored in the Quality Assurance
Department to ensure that the information is considered to be of a peer
review nature. These recommendations were communicated forcefully
throughout the educational process of piloting and implementing the
Occurrence Screen system.

Without a doubt, the most important element contributing to the success
of this process was the time spent working with physicians and hospital

departments to gain their support. As previously indicated, the directors of Quality Assurance and Risk Management met individually with many physicians and department heads and representatives, in addition to attending numerous medical staff committee and department meetings.

Another significant aspect of the process was the obstacle faced by the directors of Risk Management and Quality Assurance in trying to convey an understanding of the correct use of the multipart form. As stated earlier, directions on completion and routing of the form were included on the back of the form. This reminded less frequent users of the form of the use and flow of information and also served as a means of education for new users.

Another important part of this process was the development of the reporting capability of the system. The primary objective was to develop a computer program that would provide reports based on any aspect of information collected. Prior to the pilot, the directors of Risk Management and Quality Assurance consulted with a university graduate student who had a computer background to formalize the objectives of the reporting capability. More information on the resulting computer interface is presented later in this chapter.

Other decisions that the task force needed to make involved staff resources to operate and maintain a system. A decision was made to have the directors of Quality Assurance and Risk Management review every Occurrence Screen. This would serve as early warning of situations for Risk Management and provide an opportunity for Quality Assurance to review the type of information screened. After the group discussed the potential amount of information that could be generated and reflected on its desire to provide feedback to staff in a timely manner, it was decided that hiring a half-time staffperson to serve as a data manager would be necessary.

Pilot

The Occurrence Screen pilot consisted of using the form on five units that were representative of the institution: a surgical unit, a medical unit, a combined medical-surgical unit, an intensive care unit, and the Emergency Department (included upon the request of the Emergency Department staff and physician chairman of the Emergency Department Quality Assurance Committee). The Emergency Department physicians were obviously enthusiastic and supportive of the concept. After one month of staff education, including Nursing, Pharmacy, and all other involved departments, the pilot was initiated and conducted for a one-month period.

During the pilot, daily rounds on the units were conducted jointly by the directors of Risk Management and Quality Assurance to continue educating, answering questions, and providing feedback to staff. During the first week, rounds occurred at various times in the day in order to contact employees on all shifts.

Subsequently, an evaluation of the pilot was completed. The response was positive, with the staff reporting the following:

1. The form was easy to use.
2. Staff welcomed the ability to communicate interdepartmentally at the time of reporting an occurrence without duplicating their documentation.
3. Staff strongly supported replacing the previous three forms with one form.
4. Staff remained confused about the routing of the multipart form, particularly who to send the copies to in each department. A routing guide was developed to address this problem.
5. Staff were eager to use reports generated by this system in various ways (in Quality Assurance activities, etc.).

Staff members also provided the task force with a number of worthwhile suggestions regarding form design and directions. This feedback was reported to the Quality Evaluation and Review Committee for final approval. Unanimous support was received to proceed with the new form's implementation.

In preparation for hospital-wide implementation, extensive education was conducted; it included the following:

- presenting the Occurrence Screen system to all pertinent medical staff committees, such as the Pharmacy and Therapeutics Committee, the Ambulatory Care Committee, the Dietary Committee, and the Infection Control Committee
- meeting individually with large departments (i.e., Nursing and Pharmacy)
- presenting the Occurrence Screen at house staff/resident meetings
- presenting the system to hospital managers at regularly scheduled "management briefings"
- providing education sessions for all hospital and clinic staff
- presenting the Occurrence Screen system to administrators at an "Administrative Council" meeting
- publishing an article summarizing the system in the hospital training and education newsletter

- distributing via paychecks individual letters from the Hospital Super-intendent and Director of Clinical Affairs to all faculty, house staff, and hospital staff, describing the system and its implementation

Implementation

Implementation occurred on May 2, 1988. During the first two weeks of implementation, daily rounds at multiple times were again conducted on all in-patient units and clinics. In addition, the Quality Assurance and Risk Management directors were available to provide further education and follow-up on specific questions to departments, clinics, nursing units, and so on. To this day, rounds continue to occur approximately twice per month for follow-up on issues such as the appropriateness of form use and form completion and its routing. This frequent personal contact is believed to be a major factor in the success of the program. After six months of use, the results of this Occurrence Screen system were as follows:

1. Increased reporting: More than twice as many Occurrence Screens as incident reports are being received. Staff are more aware of quality issues overall.
2. Increased information: Much information that was not collected pre-viously is now available. For example, increased reporting of medi-cation errors has occurred, reporting of equipment and supply problems now occurs, and follow-up for department heads is pro-vided.
3. More complete forms: Users have indicated that the Ocurrence Screen is much easier to fill out than the previous incident reports.
4. Positive feedback: Users prefer the current system of problem iden-tification and reporting. Furthermore, those reporting have not ex-pressed a fear of punitive actions.
5. Increase in physicians reporting: Although a relatively small per-centage of reports are initiated by physicians, in the past none were.
6. Continued informal reporting: This remains a strong link between medical and/or hospital staff and Risk Management. An Occurrence Screen is completed by Risk Management or Quality Assurance as a result of a telephone call or note regarding an occurrence, so that information can be entered into the database.

Overall, it is felt that the success of the system is primarily attributable to the simplicity of the use of the Occurrence Screen, the form's design, and the combination of three reporting mechanisms into one. After a six-month evaluation, a report was presented to the Quality Evaluation and Review Committee. The committee, along with the staff, continues to view this system positively.

Report Capability

As with any system, management of the information generated is paramount to the success of the Occurrence Screen. The potential for large amounts of information being reported was recognized early in the process. For this reason plans to develop a computer-based data management system were initiated prior to the pilot and implementation.

A decision was made to utilize a stand-alone microcomputer system rather than to attempt to link with the hospital's mainframe. This decision was based on the task force's objectives:

1. Ensure data integrity: The hospital information system did not collect information to the level of specificity needed.
2. Maintain confidentiality of the information: Limited access to the information had to be ensured.
3. Expedite system development: The hospital information system would likely have been unable to meet necessary time frames or to provide the flexibility required.

Based on previous successful experience with dBase III-Plus in the Quality Assurance and Risk Management departments, it was decided to utilize this software for the system. As an extension of the philosophy that had guided the Occurrence Screen's development, it was felt that the means of information input and update and report generation needed to be simple and flexible. Attempts to meet user needs for simplified data entry and report generation were recognized. For that reason, data input follows the flow of the form and is based on recognized and standardized hospital abbreviations, terminology, and the like. Input includes

- "demographic" information (patient and occurrence; see Exhibit 6-1, Part I)
- identification of the respective occurrence (see Exhibit 6-1, Part II)
- summarization of the occurrence and consequences of the occurrence (i.e., permanent or temporary injury, death, no consequence), including the extent of any treatment required (see Exhibit 6-1, Parts III and IV)
- follow-up action (see Exhibit 6-1, Part V)

Numerous reports can be requested for various time frames. For example, monthly, quarterly, annual, or user-specific interval reports on specific occurrence types, occurrence locations, departments involved, physicians involved, in-patient or clinic service specific detail, and summary reports are available. In addition, the Pharmacy and Therapeutics Committee, the Quality Evaluation and Review Committee, and the Nursing Quality of Care Committee all receive specifically designated reports. Thus far, users are satisfied and in some cases overwhelmed with their respective reports. This is because of the extent and type of information available and the fact that many of those now receiving reports never received formal reports or formal feedback through the incident report or the less-than-effective service report.

It is recognized that enhancements of the various reports may be necessary to meet user needs. This will be feasible and quite simple due to the nature of dBase III-Plus. Basically, any information input can serve as a selection parameter or report element. In addition, reports correlating occurrences with diagnosis, length of stay, age, and so forth, if desired, will be feasible because of select data elements already included in the system.

Once again, simplicity, flexibility, and an eye on the users were the guidelines utilized in the software development, just as was true in all other facets of the system's design and implementation. It is felt that within the next six months, the system can be refined to the greatest extent possible, in an attempt to meet user needs.

As stated throughout this chapter, what was presented and implemented as a simple, complementary process to be used as a basis for problem identification and peer review has proven quite successful at UWHC. It is believed that this or a similar system can successfully be implemented in most health care facilities.

NOTES

1. Kathleen N. Lohr, Karl D. Yordy, and Samuel O. Thier, "Current Issues in Quality of Care Evaluation," *Health Affairs* (Spring 1988): 5–18.

2. William Jessee, "Perspectives," *Hospital Peer Review* 6, no. 3 (Mar. 1981): 28–29.

3. Ganson Purcell, Jr., "Quality Assurance/Utilization Management and Risk Management: Deterrents to Professional Liability," *Clinical Obstetrics and Gynecology* 31, no. 1 (Mar. 1988).

4. Joint Commission on Accreditation of Healthcare Organizations, *Accreditation Manual for Hospitals*, Chicago: Joint Commission, 1988.

Occurrence Screen Policy 4.22

I. PURPOSE

Prompt and accurate reporting of a patient or visitor occurrence assures complete documentation of the facts and the necessary follow-up related to an occurrence. All occurrences are reviewed to determine whether a patient or visitor requires immediate assistance, to support hospital and medical staff peer review activities through all quality assurance committees, to prevent a recurrence, to improve the quality of patient care, and to determine whether there may be a liability risk.

II. POLICY

An Occurrence Screen form must be completed whenever there is an occurrence involving a patient or visitor that is not consistent with the accepted routine operation of the hospital or the routine care of a particular patient or is an unusual or unexpected response by the patient to standard treatment or medical intervention. Documentation of occurrences is essential to facilitate peer review, identify internal problems, or respond to possible liability matters. These forms should be initiated immediately and processed within 24 hours of the occurrence. The form must not be duplicated, to ensure protection under the Wisconsin Peer Review Statute, Section 146.38. Questions concerning this policy should be referred to the Director of Quality Assurance or the Coordinator of Risk Management.

III. FORMS USED

Occurrence Screen, UWHC Form #453

Source: Courtesy of University of Wisconsin Hospital and Clinics, Madison, Wisconsin.

IV. PROCEDURE
  A. The Occurrence Screen is considered a peer review document and is to be utilized for all occurrences involving patients that represent known or potential medical or system problems or situations. Forms are to be completed promptly to allow for review and follow-up by all parties involved or affected.
  B. If a visitor is involved in an occurrence and is injured, the visitor should be referred to the Emergency Department for evaluation by medical personnel; the referral and its acceptance or refusal must be recorded on the Occurrence Screen.
  C. Sections I through III are to be completed by the hospital employee or medical staff member who identified the occurrence. The written description of the occurrence (Section III) should include only factual statements describing the incident and the patient's condition, i.e., what as a matter of fact happened, excluding speculation and assignment of fault.
  D. As pertinent, the physician (or other health professional, as appropriate) reviews the form and then completes and signs Section IV of the form as soon as she or he has seen and evaluated the patient.
  E. Once the "statement of occurrence" (Section IV) is completed, the respective supervisor reviews and follows up on the occurrence. A summary of the follow-up is recorded in Section V. The supervisor then separates the forms by sending the white copy to the Quality Assurance office (as directed on the form), the yellow copy to the designated reviewer of the form for his or her department, and the pink copy to the designated contact in the other department involved in the occurrence. If no other department is involved in the occurrence, the pink copy remains attached to the yellow copy.

  Ultimately, all copies are to be forwarded to the Quality Assurance office where a central file is maintained. Forms are shared with the Coordinator for Risk Management for review. Persons performing final review in each of the respective departments should sign the bottom of the form ("reviewed" line). Photocopies of the form should not be made, to ensure protection of these forms under the Wisconsin Peer Review Statute.
  F. Summaries and, as necessary, detailed reports of Occurrence Screens will be regularly presented, reviewed, and acted upon by all responsible departments through their quality assurance activities. In addition, the Quality Evaluation and Review Com-

mittee and other medical staff and hospital committees will receive reports and conduct review of specific cases or trends identified. Action will then be taken to resolve the problem(s) and to ensure that subsequent follow-up occurs.

G.   The Associate Superintendent or the Coordinator of Risk Management should be notified immediately by telephone of occurrences of a serious nature resulting in severe or permanent injury or death, or of occurrences that require immediate resolution while the patient is still hospitalized, such as need for further medical care or a lengthened hospital stay. The Associate Superintendent and/or Coordinator of Risk Management will discuss all occurrences of a serious nature that may have liability implications with the attorney for the Center for Health Sciences and the Director of Clinical Affairs.

V.   COORDINATION
Ann Mansfield, Coordinator of Risk Management
Eileen Smith, Associate Superintendent
Linnea Wiseman, Director of Quality Assurance
Quality Evaluation and Review Committee

chapter 7

The Importance of Staff Education as a Risk Management Tool

Sandra L. Jesser

INTRODUCTION

This chapter is designed to provide risk managers and other members of the health care team who are responsible for risk management education with the basic principles and concepts involved in developing and implementing the educational component of the risk management process.

THE ROLE OF THE RISK MANAGER AS EDUCATOR

Risk management is an information- and education-based system. In most organizations, the need for risk management education is ongoing, and the opportunities to provide risk management education are endless.

The risk manager is key in directing and developing risk management educational programs. Staff education is one of the most important elements of a health care risk management program, since it provides the foundation for effective risk control and loss prevention.

In many situations, education will begin with defining risk management for the organization. Because of the different philosophies and organizational structures involved in health care facilities (and the way they tend to become more complex with size) and the various backgrounds of persons in risk management positions, the design of risk management programs can vary considerably.

The risk manager, as the recognized expert in the field, will be expected to define the risk management process. Included in this definition will be the scope of services to be provided and the various functions of the risk management department for the organization. These concepts will be based on the goals and objectives of senior management and the overall operational plan of the facility.

Conceptually, most departments in a hospital or medical center will have some general understanding of risk management. However, it may not be totally accurate, is often incomplete, and may not incorporate recent changes and developments. Therefore, a prime responsibility of the risk manager is to identify pre-existing conceptions and then to communicate a thorough understanding of the process to all departments by applying the technical body of risk management information to the activities of each department. In this way, the risk manager and department managers can utilize their individual expertise to effectively manage risk exposures. The risk manager supplies technical assistance and methodology; the operational manager supplies expertise in the particular department's activities.

GOALS AND OBJECTIVES OF RISK MANAGEMENT EDUCATION

Risk management education is, first, one of the best ways to introduce governing boards, advisory committees, medical staffs, administrators, and other members of the organization to both the need and the value of risk management. Second, an effective program requires continuous support and commitment and must involve the participation of all departments. A third goal of risk management education is to positively influence the quality of patient care by providing feedback and quality of care information to all departments. This information may prevent and/or reduce the frequency and severity of those incidents and accidental losses that result in costly claim settlements and lawsuits. Finally, risk management education endeavors to teach all members of the health care team to incorporate risk management principles and considerations into the decision-making process so that direct patient care and other related services can be successfully defended when challenged in the courtroom.

The success of any risk management program depends to a large degree on the credibility of the risk manager. Risk managers who spend the majority of their time behind a desk or sequestered in an office will find the necessary support, commitment, and participation in their organization to be at a low level. Visibility translates into credibility and accessibility when risk managers take the lead in presenting the majority of routine and ongoing educational programs. If you have staff responsible for critical components of the risk management program, such as the claims analyst or someone primarily managing the incident reporting system, the quality assurance liaison, and other program assistants, it is just as important that these persons have exposure in the organization. Many forums lend themselves well to an introduction of the risk management team and a brief presentation from each team member on his or her area of responsibilty. This sends a strong message that risk management is taken seriously, demonstrates the supportive and service elements of the program, and encourages participation. All of the risk management department's functions can be associated with the persons performing them.

Setting Up the Education Process

Many hospitals have formal, organized education departments. In situations where a centralized education department exists, risk management programs can be coordinated with it. (Furthermore, in institutions where nursing, medical, or technology schools exist, efforts should be made to provide instruction on those aspects of course curriculum relating to the management of risk and the maintenance of quality.)

There are many advantages to developing these relationships. Education departments are an excellent resource for the novice risk manager, or even for an experienced one who needs assistance in developing educational presentations. The education department can help in writing educational objectives, organizing material, developing effective audiovisual aids, arranging for an appropriate classroom, advertising the program, and arranging for taping of the presentation for repeated use. Most important, however, is the fact that risk management education usually qualifies for continuing education credit for physicians, nurses, and many other licensed health care providers. In some states, a certain number of continuing education credits in risk management are required in order to maintain one's license to practice, which may provide staff with additional incentive to attend risk management education programs. The education department has the mechanism in place to approve programs for continuing education credit and to issue certificates of attendance serving as proof of continuing education. There are specific guidelines educational programs must meet to qualify for continuing education credit. The education department can ensure that these guidelines are met and assist with any paperwork. Usually, minimal work is required on the part of the risk manager. Exhibit 7-1 is a standard outline for designing an educational program.

Exhibit 7-1 Sample Form for Designing Educational Programs/Inservices

Program Date
_____

Title of Presentation
_____

Forum/Group/Target Audience
_____

Name of Speaker(s)
_____

_____

General Outline of Presentation
_____

_____

_____

Educational Objectives
_____

_____

_____

Submitted by   *Date*
_____

Planning Presentations

Program and presentation planning must coordinate several different elements, including

- topic
- forum
- time
- method of presentation

These elements are not independent of one another and must be carefully selected to meet the needs of each particular program. A good topic presented to the wrong group without adequate time will defeat the purpose and possibly turn the audience off to the process. Not all topics can be presented in the same way, and changing the format of programs often helps to maintain the interest of the audience. Fortunately for the risk manager working in a health care facility, the availability of topics, forums, and methods of presentation will not be a problem. Time commitments can be more difficult, especially in a large medical center or a teaching institution, but programs can be tailored for whatever time frame departments can schedule. Lectures can also be taped so that they may be viewed by those working on "off-shifts." There are also many opportunities for unplanned, spontaneous programs.

Topics

Topics should always be current and relevant to the audience. Random risk management education is rarely effective unless it is combined with information of current concern to the audience. The topic must be one the audience group perceives to be critical to its practice or function, or specific, readily identified problems and/or issues within the institution. It is always a good idea to coordinate programs with a key person in the department who can assist in the identification of specific issues or areas of concern. Much general risk management information can be included along with a focused topic, and the program can be tailored to applications that are practical and meaningful to the group. Appropriate topics for risk management programs may include the following:

- overview of the risk management program, including the formal risk management policy of the organization, goals and objectives of the program, scope of services, hospital staff with authority and responsibility for risk management, and reporting relationships (especially appropriate for new employees)
- incident reporting or occurrence screening (most hospitals have one or the other or a combination of both), with emphasis on the need for staff to complete these appropriately and the feedback that will result
- specific closed cases, with a discussion of the risk management issues involved
- communication skills
- documentation requirements
- management and follow-up of a serious incident, including disclosure discussions with patients and families
- description of the professional liability coverage for the hospital, including claims-handling procedures

- presentation of a mock trial
- confidentiality and privacy issues
- informed consent and informed refusal issues
- ethical issues and their risk management implications
- appropriate handling of patient complaints
- release of information from the medical record
- subpoenas, summons, and complaints and other legal correspondence
- current critical issues in health care, for example, nursing shortage issues, AIDS-related issues, and federal regulatory concerns

The above list is not all-inclusive but includes the most common topics that can be expected in most risk management education programs. Some of these topics are complex and best presented individually. Others can be combined, depending on the amount of time scheduled for a presentation.

Forums/Target Audiences

Just as there are a number of topics on risk management issues that can be the basis of an educational program, hospitals, large medical centers, and other health care organizations present a number of forums. This variety of forums provides an excellent opportunity for the risk manager to teach risk management skills at all levels of the organization and to educate staff on a variety of current risk management issues. Some of these include the following:

- orientations for new employees, physicians, and nurses (faculty and house staff orientations in a teaching facility or university setting)
- committee meetings
- medical staff case presentation meetings
- mortality and morbidity conferences
- grand rounds (medical and nursing)
- nursing unit staff meetings
- departmental staff meetings
- various administrative forums, such as monthly or quarterly department head meetings, hospital management council, and board meetings
- one-on-one or individual requests for consultation
- formal continuing education programs and other meetings set up primarily for education

Scheduling time for risk management education as a part of the above meetings can be a two-way initiative. Many times a spokesperson from a particular group will request that someone from risk management present a topic of interest or issue at a particular meeting. For the most part, the risk manager will need to do some aggressive marketing of the value and availability of risk management education, to begin generating some of these invitations. Initially, most risk managers will have to take the lead and contact key persons within the various groups and forums in the organization and request time on their agendas. This is where it becomes important, once again, to select the topic carefully, identifying the needs of the group and the amount of time for the presentation. Limit the scope of initial presentations to one or two key concepts. Risk management is not necessarily an area in which the majority of health care personnel feel comfortable participating. Confidence in the risk manager and the credibility of the program and an appreciation for the risk management function may develop slowly. Attempting to impart the total body of technical risk management information to clinically oriented groups will be fatal to the program, as well as to the learning process.

Time

The length of time for a presentation can vary, from ten minutes for an orientation program to six to eight hours for an all-day seminar or conference. There is a wide range between these two extremes; the final time length selected should accommodate the various forums previously described. If the forum is primarily an educational meeting, as many case presentation meetings and staff meetings are today, the risk manager may find the entire time devoted to the topic or issue selected, and a comprehensive, in-depth discussion can take place. These generally are about 45 minutes to one hour in length and always involve participation of the group. On the other hand, most orientation schedules are packed with presentations from many areas of the organization. Time constraints prohibit providing anything but the most general information, and usually only a few minutes (5 to 15) are scheduled for each presenter. (When this is the case, it is helpful to provide handouts to reinforce the information presented.) The main purpose of an orientation presentation is to provide exposure, to associate a service with a person in the organization, rather than to give a lot of detail; due to the volume of information included in orientations, detailed information is rarely retained.

The important consideration for the risk management professional is to be willing to provide information applicable to any request and to have a good overview-type program established, which can be condensed or expanded as necessary. Never turn down an opportunity to meet with a group in the organization. Not only will there be a direct effect on the group receiving the presentation, but also one may hope that news related to the presentation will be passed onto other groups. Each group that participates in risk management education is then in a position to assist in educating others when the same issue comes up in another setting. The more contacts risk management has within an organization, the greater the likelihood that there will be someone knowledgeable on the scene when an event occurs that requires notification of risk management or intervention by the risk manager. This greatly increases the opportunity for risk management to be involved in a timely, proactive manner, thereby increasing the effectiveness of the risk management program.

Method of Presentation

The last element in planning presentations relates to the method of presentation. As with topics, forums, and time frames, there are a number of methods to choose from, and not all are appropriate for every situation. The method used will also depend on the size of the group and its level of knowledge on the subject. The purpose of the particular forum and the time allowed for presentation must also be considered. There are both *formal* and *informal* methods of presentation. A brief review of the more useful methods for each category follows.

Among the formal methods of presentation, the *lecture method* is one of the most widely used. This method is particularly useful when the group lacks content background and is the best way to present new information. Maximum information can be provided in minimum time, and while it can be used for any group size, it is probably the most effective method for large groups where individual participation is usually limited. A disadvantage to the lecture method is that lecturing is not a natural or easy skill for all risk managers. It is always a good idea to enhance lectures with visual aids, where possible, to clarify or simplify major points. Maintaining audience interest by using examples from the group's point of reference is also helpful. Lecture presentations should always allow for a brief question and answer period at the end. The types of questions asked will give the risk manager or other presenter some measure of how successfully the information was received. The lecture method is commonly utilized either alone or in conjunction with other methods for seminars and continuing education programs that are at least an hour or more in length. In this and all other methods, it is helpful to provide a written outline of the discussion prior to the lecture and a written summary of the content presented after the lecture.

The *discussion method* is used primarily for problem solving. Risk managers should use the discussion method of presentation in the meetings of committees that they are members of or that have asked them to attend to specifically represent the risk management perspective. This method is oriented to individuals in a group. Participation, involvement, and inter-action are characteristics of discussion, and the process is generally one of examining issues and making decisions. Discussion is not suitable for com-plex content, for this reason: It can be easy for discussion to stray from the topic or issue. Time can be wasted if committee members have not prepared for the topic, so it is always appropriate to provide background material and other resource information, as well as specific questions to the members, prior to the meeting. This will involve contacting the person chairing the committee and submitting material in time for its inclusion on the agenda. The discussion method is also appropriate for many unit or department staff meetings, which can include problem solving as well as information sharing.

The *case study method* is really a variation of the discussion method. In health care this generally occurs at case presentation meetings initiated or planned specifically for this purpose. Programs utilizing this method can be presented well with a team approach. The medical aspects of the case can be presented by the health care practitioner, and the risk management points can be presented or reviewed by the risk manager. The focus of the case study method is to look at a specific case or problem and follow it through to a conclusion. Other forums that may utilize this method are mortality and morbidity conferences, various peer review committees, and most medical and nursing grand rounds programs. In order to be effective as an educational technique, the case method must be directed at the group that, professionally and technically, shares the background knowledge and expertise to integrate the various concepts presented. Case study presen-tations usually stimulate high levels of participation by various members of the group and are very adaptable to individual needs, facilitating the sharing of different and even controversial viewpoints. Since this method is one that most health care practitioners are familiar with, it can be very successfully used by a well-prepared risk manager.

Programmed instruction and *self-study learning modules* are other tech-niques available for incorporation into educational programs or for use alone. These include formats such as audiotapes or videotapes with post-tests and/or workbooks, workbooks or study guides with a test, and various home study courses that may include textbook or combined media. Most people like things they can do at their leisure, and this is a helpful method of accommodating the busy schedules of health care professionals. The advantage for the risk management professional is the ability to develop the program once, duplicate it, and have it available all of the time and at multiple locations. Programs can be customized to a specific audience and personalized to a particular organization. The major disadvantage is that unless there is some incentive involved, the programs tend simply to collect dust. To avoid such a fate, it would be particularly good to coordinate these methods with the education department so that risk management programs would be in the distribution schedule along with other professional and clinical topics for continuing education.

Whatever the method of presentation, it is always advantageous to consider the ways in which people learn. Listening is only one way. Many people learn by reading, and just about anyone can learn visually. As much as possible, presentations should include appropriate visual aids, such as slides and overhead transparencies. Handout material is also a good reinforcement. Not only does it give participants something to take with them, but if properly designed it will also provide space for meaningful notes and become a valuable reference tool later on.

Thus far the discussion has been directed at formal methods of presentation. There are many informal methods as well. Some of these include the various interhospital communiqués, memos, and so forth, in which risk management issues can be addressed; the establishment of a risk management newsletter (a medical staff letter would be an especially good one); bulletins and information sheets that address specific risk management questions, which can be sent as follow-ups after a telephone consultation; telephone consultations; and distributions to staff of selected articles from the journals and periodicals found in most risk managers' professional reading.

While it is not within the scope of this text to present an in-depth review of all the techniques and various aspects of adult education, in planning risk management presentations it is important to keep in mind some of the basic principles involved for working with the adult learner. Not all methods are appropriate, since they are not all flexible enough to accommodate the busy schedules and lifestyles of working professionals in the fast-paced and relatively stressful environment of a large hospital, medical center, or clinic.

Physicians, nurses, and other health care providers do not like having their time wasted. They learn from others' experience as well as their own, see themselves as independent, need to see the results of what has been learned, have definite thoughts regarding authority, have ideas to contribute, and must be provided mechanisms that encourage participation in the process. Information must be relevant. Educational programs, to be successful and effective, must address issues related to the work situation, include topics of special interest to the group, present information on areas perceived by the group to be problems, relate to a current or recent happening that has stimulated action and raised awareness, and, most of all, must be reality oriented. Programs that present a particular situation, the major facts, and the action or behavior required are generally well received. This utilizes the formal time maximally and gives busy health care professionals time to assimilate content, think it through, and practice the skills taught. It is persisting changes in actions and behavior that confirm that learning has been achieved. Programs that are too long or too technical will not change practice.

The resource list at the end of this chapter contains several references on educational program planning that provide additional, more detailed information for the risk manager wanting to review or to increase knowledge and skill in this area.

Presentation/Program Files

An excellent method of storing presentations for easy retrieval and use is to keep all the material together in a three-ring vinyl binder with inside pockets. Slides can be stored in $8\frac{1}{2}$-by-11-inch, three-hole-punched, vinyl slide protectors. Overhead transparencies, with a sheet of plain white paper between them to keep them from adhering to one another, will fit in the inside pocket of the binder's cover. Include any handout material too; it will then be available for quick duplication. Maintained as a part of the risk management department library, such binders keep educational materials ready for use when needed.

Aids to the Process

Setting up the Educational Calendar

A schedule of presentations for the annual educational calendar is probably the most common way of formalizing education in most hospitals. While some risk management programs can be done this way (i.e., new employee orientation), many others need more flexibility in scheduling to be effective. Scheduling a quarterly program on incident reporting may seem reasonable, but it may have limited attendance and may not be able to maintain a high priority as time pressures and priorities change.

Risk management education is more effectively scheduled by determining content and target areas, rather than number of programs per month each calendar year. A more realistic objective would be to provide a risk management in-service to each major department sometime during the year and to schedule departments each month so that there is always a target audience, rather than scheduling programs each month and hoping staff will show up.

There are several core programs that should always be current and available for presentation. These include

• overview of the risk management program and process

- incident reporting
- claims management procedures
- insurance coverage

These programs are designed to answer the basic and routine questions that are often asked of risk managers, such as

- What is risk management?
- What does the hospital's program do?
- When do I report an incident?
- What are examples of reportable incidents?
- What do I do if I am sued?

Special or topic-specific programs can be developed as needed or requested and can be used alone or in conjunction with any combination of core programs.

Risk Management Manual

A risk management manual is an extremely useful educational tool. A well-organized manual should contain the risk management statement or plan, policies and procedures for the function of the risk management department, and guidelines that outline steps to be taken in certain situations (e.g., follow-up after a serious incident or steps in preparing proceedings for court-ordered consent and other similarly complex issues that require continuity in their management and assurance that sequential steps have been completed). Many of the guidelines appropriate for a manual can be produced in a checklist format (see Exhibit 7-2) and used at the time information is collected. The risk manager can then be confident that information has been collected in a systematic manner and that the chance of something critical being missed is greatly reduced.

Risk management is not static. The body of knowledge maintained by the risk manager and members of the risk management department must be continually updated. Changes in the law that affect health care practice, new programs and services the organization develops, standards and code changes, technological advancement, and myriad overlapping ethical and legal issues will affect the risk picture and require the risk manager to reassess and revise risk management procedures and protocol. Much education takes place within the risk management department itself, to keep current with the developments in the field and to maintain an effective program. At least on an annual basis, the risk management manual should be reviewed for accuracy and revised to reflect any changes.

Exhibit 7-2 Risk Management Checklist for Follow-Up Information—Serious Incidents

☐ Name, age, diagnosis, and prognosis of the patient.
☐ Basic description of what happened.
☐ Names of caregivers involved (will want to talk with them before they leave their shift).
☐ Specific outcome/injury and whether or not it was a direct result of the incident.
☐ Is the attending physician present? Been notified? Who has the best rapport/relationship with the patient or family?
☐ What family members are present? Are more anticipated? (Sometimes it is best to wait until all are present before anyone talks to the family or to designate a contact person so that information is consistent and controlled.)
☐ Has anyone talked with patient or family? If so, what were they told?
☐ Any equipment involved? (Should be sequestered and referred to clinical engineering for inspection.)
☐ Medication error? (Syringes or containers should be saved for analysis.)
☐ Instruction on communication with patient and family given by risk management.
☐ Instruction on documentation in medical record given by risk management.
☐ Incident report completed.
☐ Claims management personnel, insurance representative, or hospital attorney notified.

Other useful information to include in the risk management manual are various resource lists, such as telephone numbers and mailing addresses of key personnel in the organization meeting frequently with the risk management department; professional organizations and agencies; defense counsel and names of key contact persons; and books, periodicals, and reference lists for selected risk management topics and general information.

All forms used by risk management should be included in the manual with guidelines for their completion.

Used as a reference for risk management personnel, the manual provides a consistent method for managing both routine and complex risk management issues. It is an excellent tool to orient new employees to the risk management department and a useful resource for persons providing administrative on-call duty for the organization. Selected policies and procedures from the manual, providing general information and directions applicable for all departments of the organization (such as the policy of incident reporting), should also be included in the hospital's general policy and procedure manual.

Utilizing Other Staff Members

The risk management department should remain the focal point for all risk management functions and the teaching of risk management skills and risk control. However, risk management education should involve other resources both internal and external to the organization.

Available external resources include defense counsel, claims management personnel (if claims are not handled internally), insurance agency representatives and educators, and other risk managers. Outside professionals should be chosen carefully. Make sure their philosophy of risk management is compatible with the risk management program at your institution and that it will serve as reinforcement for that program. The risk manager should also maintain the primary role as educator and coordinate all risk management educational programs.

In many cases, risk managers have developed programs that are not necessarily unique to their organizations but that address a particular issue. Networking among peer risk managers from other hospitals and health care agencies can generate a comprehensive list of programs and presenters, and risk managers can take advantage of this available expertise and offer their own by exchanging guest presentations with other hospitals. Drawing on the expertise of outside professionals can significantly contribute to the education component of the risk management program.

Many persons involved in risk management functions may not be formal members of the risk management department but may nevertheless serve as internal educational resources. Some of these are patient representatives, infection control committee members, the biomedical engineer, the fire and safety officer, the disaster coordinator, legal counsel, and social services providers. There are many opportunities to present joint programs with these people, and this is a good way to promote the active involvement of staff in risk management. Including other staff in educational programs shows an understanding of the particular problems in that area, allows for different and unusual viewpoints to be presented, and encourages the introduction of specific expertise from persons who can elaborate on department-related situations and provide meaningful examples.

IN-SERVICE EDUCATION

Providing in-service to staff and new employees is very important. It is always easier to teach the right way initially than to facilitate an unlearning and retraining process later. In-service needs are sometimes recognized and programs requested by the department head, but in many situations determining in-service needs will require the acute intuition of the risk manager. An interesting phenomenon about risk management is that there are just about as many perceptions of what it constitutes as there are people. And like the six blind men all touching different parts of the elephant, all these views are individually right but jointly very wrong. In addition, it is a growing, changing field, developing rapidly as a distinct discipline. Risk management professionals may have a variety of backgrounds, including law, medicine, nursing, medical records, quality assurance, safety, insurance, and business and finance. It is not too surprising that risk management programs can differ considerably from organization to organization.

It is easy to get a reading on the in-service needs of specific departments as well as the organization's concept of risk management by carefully listening to the kinds of questions being asked in meetings and other forums and by studying the nature of the calls received in the risk management department. If they are not appropriately managed within the scope of the risk management process, you can be sure there are some educational deficits and gaps regarding that process. These gaps should be the focal point of the risk manager's program development. Correcting these deficits will help the risk manager build credibility, as well as establish the parameters for the risk management program. In-service programs for staff and new employees should define the risk management process and teach basic risk management skills. These include communication, documentation, incident reporting, and loss control techniques, and how to apply these skills to the specific department or area.

Educating the Professional Staff

Physicians, nurses, and other health care providers are experts in their particular areas of practice. The purpose of risk management education for professional staff is to teach risk management skills and assist staff in developing a clear understanding of the risk management process so that effective risk control can take place. As this process becomes a part of each health care provider's practice, risk management concerns and considerations become a natural part of the decision-making process.

A review of the risk management process, emphasizing communication and documentation requirements, can positively influence the risk management effort. Whatever else may be involved in a patient complaint or an actual claim, it is certain that anger, frustration, and dissatisfaction are always be basic ingredients. Many problems arise out of the quality and tone of communications and the quality and volume of documentation. Inflammatory remarks, incomplete documentation (including missing or altered documentation), statements that point the finger at peers or colleagues, departmental infighting, statements not related to the care of the patient, and inappropriate or derogatory abbreviations that require little imagination on the part of patients or their attorneys to interpret are samples of communication and documentation that can be most damaging.

Much has been written describing many other problems encountered when communication breakdowns occur and the perceptions of the patient are different from those of the physician or nurse. The importance of listening to patients and making sure explanations are thorough and in language easily understood cannot be emphasized enough.

Presentations to professional staff should serve to clarify the tasks and functions of risk management. Eliminate medical jargon, useless advice, and heavy-duty legal language. It is tiresome to listen to, doesn't usually impress anyone, and confuses the message since it is risk management skills and techniques the presentation should address, not law or medicine.

Documentation deficiencies will continue to be a major cause of sleepless nights for risk managers while guaranteeing success for plaintiffs' attorneys. A complete record is not necessarily a voluminous one. But many times there are notes in the record that have nothing to do with the patient's care, and some of this extraneous verbiage is actually detrimental and can be problematic when the record is reviewed for legal or other reasons.

The original purpose of the medical record was to provide a mechanism for communication between the nurse and the physician. This concept has almost been lost in the myriad of uses involving the medical record today. It is used to verify bills, provide proof of service for reimbursement, serve as evidence in a court of law, provide information for statistical studies, and the list continues. From a risk management perspective, the medical record as a communication tool needs to be re-emphasized. With this in mind, there are a few major requirements. Records must be legible, and notes should be timed, dated, and signed and should contain information and facts related to the care of the patient. Corrections are made in such a way that the original information is still visible. The most common method is by drawing a single line through the incorrect entry, writing the word "error," dating and initialing the entry, and then writing the correct information.

SPECIAL EDUCATIONAL NEEDS

Employees Involved in Lawsuits

Above and beyond general risk management educational needs, there are situations that call for special attention and instruction from the risk manager. One such situation is when professional staff members or employees are involved in a lawsuit. Most health care professionals are not comfortable dealing with anything that looks legal. Subpoenas, depositions, summons and complaints, letters of intent to sue, and phone calls from attorneys are all threatening communications that generate considerable anxiety. Staff should be told to notify risk management immediately when any kind of legal-type communication is received. The risk manager can do a lot in the way of reassuring staff and guiding them through the process. Explain to staff what can be expected, fill in any information they need to have, and ask them to review all information available related to the case. Assure them they will have representation, give them the name of the attorney who will be handling the case, and let them know their interests are being protected. It is important to instruct employees not to discuss the case with anyone except as directed by the attorney or the risk manager. Health care professionals many times do not realize that lawsuits can continue for a number of years. Explain the process to them and let them know that the risk management department is available to assist them and to answer any questions they may have at any time during the proceedings.

New Forms, Policies, and Procedures

Generally it is not the responsibility of the risk management department to develop and in-service new forms, policies, and procedures. It is, however, within the scope of risk management to assist in the development of a mechanism to ensure that in-service takes place, to review forms for content and format, and to provide input into policies and procedures that include risk management functions or require risk management action. Noncompliance with policy and procedure is a risk exposure. Until the persons responsible for implementation have been informed, it is unrealistic to expect compliance. Effective dates of policies should not be set and new forms should not be distributed until in-service is complete.

Usually, policies and procedures go through a number of revisions before they are finalized and made effective. A good way to track the various stages of review and one that increases awareness and compliance is a color-coded system telling everyone where the policy or form is in the approval process. For example, policies and forms in the "draft" stage can be printed on yellow paper, with "draft" printed clearly across the top. This sends a clear message that the item is not in effect, and the colored paper reduces the chance of its being inadvertently placed in the manual prematurely. When the form or policy is final and ready for in-service, a pink copy with a signature sheet attached should be sent out, and staff can sign when they have read the policy or reviewed the form. A time frame should be established for the in-service period, and department managers should be accountable for providing in-service in their area. And finally, a white copy to be placed in the manual, with the effective date and appropriate approval signatures, should be generated. This is a very simple, coordinated, systematic method of managing the policy, procedure, and forms development process. Until the final, signed white copy is received, the policy or procedure is still in progress. The risk management department should maintain current manuals of all organizational policies, as well as medical staff bylaws and other structural and process standards that impose a responsibility for compliance, and should receive updates as revisions are made. The risk manager should review those that have risk management involvement and recommend changes accordingly.

Awareness of Public Policy Issues

The risk manager is in a prime position to become a resource on many of the public policy issues that affect health care. Most states have addresses or numbers to call to get on mailing lists to receive copies of legislative updates. Copies of new laws passed can be obtained free of charge. Work with the hospital's legal counsel to develop a subject list they will automatically send information on when changes in the law affecting the health care system are made. Subscribe to a variety of newsletters, journals, and periodicals, and share the information generously with other areas of the organization. Participate in professional organizations and forums that address such public policy issues as HIV testing and disclosure, ethical issues, and other risk management-related information.

GUARANTEEING THAT THE PROCESS IS BENEFICIAL

The results of risk management education may not immediately result in reduced claims and lawsuits. The most immediate result will most likely be increased communication with the risk management department. This is an excellent opportunity for the risk manager to get firsthand feedback as well as to ask for input in the planning of future programs. Don't hesitate to ask staff what types of information would be most useful.

If a more formal evaluation process is desired, a simple evaluation form in a checklist format can be developed. Formal evaluations should be used with formal methods of presentation, such as lectures and seminars. Evaluations are generally required for continuing education programs. Much of the evaluation process for risk management education will be done informally. Allow for feedback after each program. Time should be adequate for questions, answers, and comments. These brief sessions will give the risk manager insight as to how the information was received by the group and whether it was processed in a useful manner. Questions and comments can be incorporated into the content of subsequent presentations. Audience feedback also stimulates more ideas and can serve as further clarification for points covered in the presentation.

Change takes place very slowly, and risk management is no exception. An increase in the number of incident reports (particularly by groups who were not reporting), an increase in requests for consultation, early involvement in follow-up of serious incidents, and early warning of potential hazards are all indications of successful risk management education that will eventually prove beneficial to the organization by reducing losses.

Risk management programs should be monitored carefully for effectiveness. Look for the subtle changes that appear only in a well-organized, systematic program, and promote these changes throughout the organization at every opportunity. Keep good statistics. Develop a method and format for reporting risk management activities to administration at least on a quarterly basis. Including statistical trending reports and various studies in this report will keep administration involved in the process and will provide a mechanism for feedback to the risk manager to ensure that risk management program development continues to reflect the overall objectives of senior and executive management and to support the general direction of the organization.

IMPORTANCE OF COOPERATION

Risk management is a staff function in most organizations even though it may appear in the line configuration on the organizational chart. Most risk managers, however, have line authority over technical risk management decisions. As a manager of a staff department, the risk manager has the staff authority to advise, recommend, and consult, rather than the line authority of the operational manager to order, command, and control.

Risk management collects information from all areas of the organization. Most information that is useful to risk managers must be provided by other departments, and the success of the program is dependent upon maintaining a centralized intelligence within the risk management department and a continuous flow of information into it. There is very little that goes on in a hospital that isn't of interest to risk management from the perspective of being able to analyze and examine the scope of activities to determine risk exposure. A high degree of coordination and cooperation must exist between operational departments and the risk management department. This becomes even more critical in teaching institutions or university settings where in addition to the routine activities of a health care organization, there are nursing students, technical training programs, and interns, residents, and fellows in the school of medicine, all participating in patient care. Risk management may also provide services to affiliated areas of a university, such as the school of dentistry and student health services.

The risk manager with staff authority has the powers of logic and persuasion as tools to obtain the necessary cooperation of other departments. Risk management must be viewed as a positive force within the organization, providing a service that assists physicians, nurses, and other health care providers. If risk management is viewed negatively as a function that only creates more work for busy professionals or as a watchdog looking over their shoulders, trying to catch them doing something wrong, the flow of information to the risk management department will be nil. On the other hand, a risk manager who is accessible, demonstrates that information will be handled confidentially, and provides useful feedback to the department will be seen as an ally, and the risk management department as a department that can be called upon for technical assistance and methodology to assist professional staff and operational managers in problem solving.

The risk manager should communicate to all departments the types of events that should initiate a call to risk management and the services available through the risk management department. It is important, however, that the risk manager and the staff of the risk management department function within the role of risk management to advise, recommend, and consult, and not become directly involved in managing the operations of a department or in solving departmental problems. This can undermine the authority and credibility of the operational manager and put the risk manager in a position of trying to implement a solution or provide direction to staff over whom the risk manager has no line authority. In addition to acting as a hindrance to problem solving rather than an assistance, it can cause additional problems for the operational department due to the risk manager's lack of expertise in the particular area. Work with the appropriate operational manager by providing the risk management perspective, not by taking over ownership of the problem or departmental operations.

Centralize the intelligence of the organization by developing cooperative, supportive relationships with administrative and operational managers, medical staff, and other personnel so that the information flow is sufficient and continuous, but decentralize the risk management functions as part of departmental decision making and problem solving.

Many times a negative attitude exists toward risk management because staff have had contact with the risk manager only when something has gone wrong or when an actual claim has been filed. Risk management has often been thought of as synonymous with claims management in the health care setting. Claims and lawsuits by their nature are negative events for most health care providers. Unfortunately, this antiquated and incomplete definition of risk management still exists in the minds of many health care providers even though the focus of risk management has changed drastically over the last decade. When the risk management department is viewed as a resource and it is clear that its activities are designed to protect the organization and the individuals that work within it, negative attitudes can change to positive ones facilitating the kind of cooperation between professional staff and the risk management department that promotes the incorporation of risk management functions into the individual practice of each health care provider.

Take the lead in letting the organization know what risk management is. Show departments what a good resource it can be. Share information in the form of constructive feedback freely, and use examples of risk prevention, risk reduction, and how proactive approaches work to reduce and eliminate serious incidents, claims, and lawsuits. There is nothing negative about prevention. An incident that didn't occur and didn't harm anyone because it was identified before it happened is very positive and hits at the heart of the risk management program. Handle information, particularly sensitive information, quietly and confidentially. Nothing will destroy the credibility of a risk manager faster than feeding risk management information into the grapevine. Protect the information other departments provide, and make sure follow-through is direct and timely so that "knee jerk" reactions are kept to a minimum and the subsequent gossip and incident enhancement that often take place are controlled or eliminated.

It is much too optimistic to assume that everyone in the organization understands the risk management process. Not only is it important for physicians, nurses, and other patient care providers to have a clear concept of this process, but also key administrative directors and department heads. The risk manager has a major responsibility to keep key persons in the organization informed of the changes and developments in risk management so that the program will receive the support needed for continued growth and ability to meet the needs of the organization.

CONCLUSION

Risk management collects information from all areas of the organization. Analysis of this information can identify risk exposure and performance deficits, which can be corrected through the development of a strong educational component in the risk management program. This is the basis of risk prevention. The risk manager is the key person in this process, but coordination with other resources both within and external to the organization is essential to the success of the program. The most useful methods of presentation are lecture, discussion, case presentation, and programmed instruction; these utilize existing meetings, committees, and other organized forums in the organization. Relevant topics and length of time for presentations as well as special educational needs are important elements to consider in developing effective educational programs.

Change will take place over a period of time. The risk management program must be continuously monitored to ensure that the process is beneficial and continues to promote the goals and objectives of the program and the organization.

REFERENCES

de Mare, George. *Communicating at the Top*. New York: John Wiley & Sons, Inc., 1968.

Doolittle, Robert J. *Professionally Speaking—A Concise Guide*. Glenview, Ill.: Professional Publishing Group, 1984.

Dyche, June. *Educational Program Development for Employees in Health Care Agencies*. Los Angeles: Tri-Oak Educational Division, 1982.

Lambert, Clark. *Secrets of a Successful Trainer—A Simplified Guide for Survival*. New York: John Wiley & Sons, Inc., 1986.

Powers, John H. *Public Speaking—The Lively Art*. Belmont, Calif.: Wadsworth Publishing Co., 1987.

Sarnoff, Dorothy, *Never Be Nervous Again*. New York: Crown Publishers, Inc., 1987.

chapter 8

The Importance of Patient Education as a Risk Management Tool

Cecelia E. Yeaton

PATIENT EDUCATION AS A COMPONENT OF RISK MANAGEMENT

Patient education is a long-standing component of health care practice. It can be as simple as verbal instructions for elevating and applying ice packs to an injured ankle, a sheet of instructions on head injury given to a motor vehicle accident patient on discharge from the emergency department, or a programmed text provided for teaching diabetics self-injection of insulin. But while patient teaching is intended as an adjunct to hands-on care, it can also be considered an adjunct to risk management. This chapter discusses the use of patient education as a means to reduce claims made against a hospital.

The present health care system in the United States often places patients in the position of coordinating services for themselves or for members of their families. Many individuals are not prepared to take on this role and are incapable of performing it appropriately or effectively. Their feelings of inadequacy will tend to govern their perceptions of the adequacy of the care that is given.

For instance, a patient who has undergone an out-patient surgery procedure will typically see the surgeon sometime in the late afternoon or early evening following the procedure. Intraoperatively, the patient may have been given an analgesic impairing his or her ability to comprehend postoperative verbal instructions on, for instance, how many days until he or she can drive a car, how soon to arrange an appointment for follow-up, and what situations require return to the hospital or immediate contact with a physician. Confusion as to appropriate follow-up precipitated by the administration of anesthesia can result in inadequate or improper aftercare resulting in injury.

The doctor or discharge staff person can give these same instructions to the patient or family member in written form. The content of this information can influence the patient's perception of the adequacy of the care given. Specifically, the more comprehensive the information provided, the better the patient (or family member) will be able to react appropriately to complications, and the better the patient will understand the recovery process. These beneficial effects will not be obtained if the written instructions do not adequately address possible postoperative problems or provide reassuring information as to the nature of the recovery period, or if they erroneously assume a high level of understanding of disease processes and treatment courses on the part of the patient. The obvious benefits to successful recovery include the patient's perception that quality care has been delivered.

The new age of health care anticipates educated consumers. One of the challenges facing risk managers is ensuring that each patient is provided the appropriate education to assist him or her in understanding the care received and the appropriateness of its outcome. Aggressive hospital marketing campaigns, coupled with media sensationalization of issues in health care, often increase a patient's expectations related to final outcome. To make these expectations more realistic requires concomitant involvement by risk management and clinical staff (nurses and physicians) in the development of an educational program to accomplish the following goals: understanding the problem or disease, understanding the treatment rendered, and recognizing that perfection is not always obtainable and that a less than perfect result does not always suggest negligence. In addition, a patient education program can be structured to provide information that will reduce patient perception of denial of access or inadequate follow-up and can assist the patient to participate in a positive manner in his or her own care.

RISK MANAGEMENT INVOLVEMENT IN PATIENT EDUCATION

Risk management professionals should become actively involved in patient education. They should meet with patient education coordinators to review topics being presented and written materials prepared for distribution to patients, in order to recommend inclusions that are appropriate from a risk management perspective.

From the risk manager's perspective, patient education that anticipates problems and provides the patient with the information to cope successfully with these problems is the ideal risk management tool. The more frequently physicians, nurses, and other caregivers provide this kind of information, the less often the patient or the family will depend on media sources or lay experts and the more often expectations will be met. Many factors must be considered in delivering effective patient education that suits risk management principles; these are laid out in Exhibit 8-1.

In the interests of good patient education and good risk management preventive measures, written patient education materials should meet the following criteria:

1. The information should be legible and written on clear, clean copies. Provide materials in translation as required by the patient population served. The information should be in simple language; avoid medical terms. Remember that the average reading level is at the seventh grade.

2. Appropriate content is critical. When explaining illness or disease, make an attempt to explain etiology, usual methods of making a diagnosis, the usual symptoms experienced, the usual treatment, and the specific follow-up treatment required. *Specific* symptoms and *specific* actions to take should be included (e.g., call the doctor, go to the emergency department, etc.). When preparing content for operative procedures, including ambulatory surgery, preoperative and postoperative materials are most effective. The preoperative material should give an explanation of the condition, its symptoms, how the diagnosis is made, what the operative procedure involves, alternatives to surgery, the expected course of recovery, and possible complications of the procedure to be performed. The postoperative information should include when to make the follow-up appointment, which symptoms should be immediately reported to the doctor during the postoperative recovery period, and the expected course of recovery.

3. Concise, thorough documentation is essential. A notation should be made in the patient care record that educational material and written or verbal instructions were given to the patient or the person responsible for the patient. A copy of the materials provided should also be kept on file, or the facility may make up forms for inclusion in the patient care record, including a self-carbon that the patient signs, acknowledging receipt of instructions.

Other risk management involvement in patient education would include risk management in-services describing the inter-relationship of risk man-

Exhibit 8-1 Sample Program on Effective Methods of Patient Education

---

I. Factors associated with patient compliance
  A. Patient characteristics
    1. health related beliefs and values
    2. psychological factors
    3. substance dependence
    4. history of noncompliance
  B. Environmental factors
    1. social support system
    2. waiting time for appointment
    3. lapse between referral and appointment
  C. Treatment factors
    1. complexity of treatment
    2. length of treatment
    3. side effects
    4. cost
    5. behavioral change component
  D. Provider-patient relationship
    1. effective transfer of information
    2. justification of need for treatment
    3. meeting patient expectations
    4. continuity of care
II. Compliance-improving activities
  A. Appointment keeping
    1. mail reminder, instructional content
    2. explanation of reason for referral to specialist
  B. Adherence to treatment
    1. verbal instructions augmented with written material, including information about possible side effects
    2. educational programs directed to specific diseases or conditions (hypertension, chronic obstructive pulmonary disease)
    3. simplification, tailoring of regimen
    4. patient involvement, self-monitoring
    5. familial support

---

agement and the patient education program and effective methods of patient education and presenting patient satisfaction surveys evaluating the effectiveness of patient education and identifying areas requiring additional education.

USE OF THE PATIENT REPRESENTATIVE OR PATIENT ADVOCATE

Patient representatives, advocates, or ombudsmen have become an important part of day-to-day hospital operation. Many hospitals have a specific guest relations department that is intended to represent the patient in situations where the patient or the family is at odds with the hospital or its staff. These patient representatives can be a valuable source of information to the risk manager not only in regard to the needs of individual patients but also in regard to common complaints, suggestions, and concerns raised by the patient or family. It is often this department that upon discharge provides the patient with a survey requesting information related to the care received during hospitalization. Generally these surveys provide a mechanism for the patient (or family member) to offer complaints or make suggestions. The hospital risk manager should plan to meet with the patient representative on a regular basis to review the surveys and to learn if there are any particular areas in the hospital that require focused attention. The patient representative—who often has a more direct relationship with patients and family members than do staff—can also describe areas where additional patient education would be most helpful.

If initiatives have been undertaken to meet identified patient needs, the risk manager should inform the patient representative of what those measures were and solicit feedback as to their success or failure.

Obviously, the ability to develop a patient education program that meets the needs of patients, their families, and the institution will depend on the ability and sensitivity of the risk manager and other hospital staff to recognize what those needs are. Once recognized, appropriate education can be of great assistance in overcoming patient complaints and preventing the lawsuits that result from patients' frustration due to lack of information and an erroneous perception of events occurring during or as a result of their hospital stay.

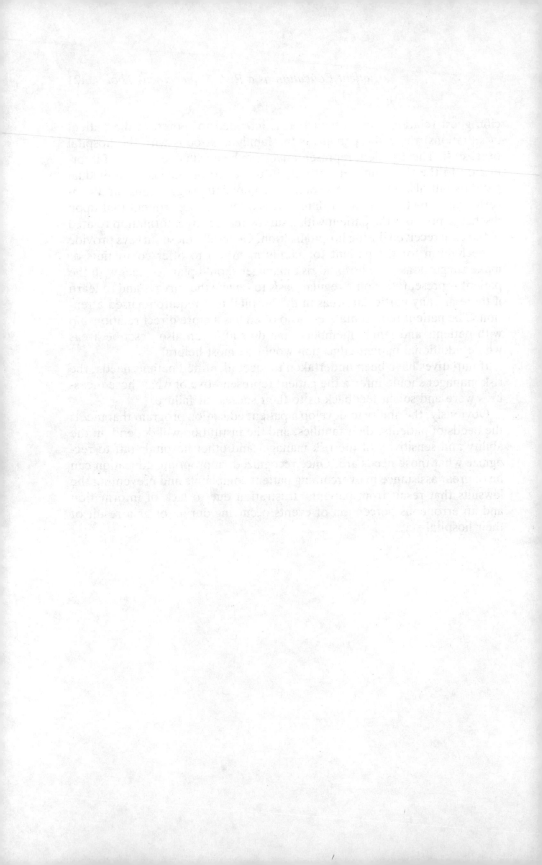

PART IV

Insurance Concepts

The first two chapters of Part IV will focus on how a risk manager determines a hospital's need to insure and the insurance options available. Chapter 9 will present information related to risk assessment—the process of quantifying the professional liability exposures facing an institution. Special emphasis will be placed on the type of data required to perform the assessment. Suggestions will also be offered on how to interpret the data. Chapter 10 will discuss the coverage options available to the hospital. Methodology to evaluate the reasonableness of excess insurance quotations will be presented as well. Following these discussions, an evaluation of the forms of insurance coverage available will be presented.

In Chapter 11 a brief overview of the insurance marketplace will be presented, along with evaluation tools with which to analyze the fiscal strength of companies. The importance of utilizing brokers and consultants when setting up an insurance program will also be discussed, and a checklist indicating important characteristics of a broker or consultant will be provided.

Chapter 12 provides additional information related to the insurance product itself. Care is taken to describe the various aspects of coverage, policy terms, and features and the common types of insurance with which the risk manager will have to become familiar.

In the final chapter of Part IV, Chapter 13, the critical element of reporting losses to the underwriter is discussed as it relates to both claims made and occurrence coverage. In order to understand the rationale for the reporting differences, an in-depth discussion of the two forms of coverage is provided. The problems of mixing these two forms of coverage are also explained. Though much of this information is very technical, understanding it is critical to ensure that the hospital is afforded appropriate coverage for all of its losses. Upon completion of this chapter, the reader should have a thorough understanding of (1) the analysis required to determine the amount and type of appropriate coverage, (2) the qualities to look for in brokers and consultants for the hospital's insurance program, (3) policy terms and features, and (4) the critical importance of complying with reporting provisions to guarantee coverage.

chapter 9

Determining the Need To Purchase Insurance

Rodney Klein
James D. Blinn

Hospital professional liability is an area of great risk. A decision on what amount of coverage to carry cannot be treated as a guessing game. Hospitals must compile comprehensive loss and exposure information and rigorously analyze the data before making the decision. This chapter will focus on two alternatives for estimating future losses with reliable precision. The first approach is a self-study technique that can be performed by the reader, while the second employs the services of a skilled professional.

INFORMATION GATHERING

Loss and exposure data must be collected, including

- Gross patient service volumes
  —in-patient days
  —out-patient visits
- Professional staff counts by service and FTEs (expressed in terms of the full-time equivalency devoted toward clinical work)
  —employed and nonemployed attending physicians
  —house staff
- Research activity (a profile of the type of research being conducted and the number of patients affected)
- Contractual obligations (indemnity agreements with vendors and other providers, transferring professional liability obligations to the hospital, e.g., house staff rotation agreements)
- Loss history

The following information is required in analyzing losses (losses being defined as both paid and reserved cases):

1. date of loss occurrence
2. description of the occurrence and injury involved
3. clinical department involved
4. dollar value of loss (both the settlement amount and other related costs)

Other related costs are defined to include fees for legal defense, expert witnesses, structured settlement specialists, court reports, and the like.

The loss history is obtained from either of two sources: risk management reserve logs or past commercial insurance carriers' loss summaries. At least seven years of loss data are required, given the infrequency of litigated professional liability claims, to establish a loss pattern.

LOSS PROJECTIONS

Future losses must be estimated. The following three steps may be used to accomplish this goal.

Step 1

Determine the expected frequency and magnitude of losses. The nature of the injury sustained is the best predictor of the value of a loss. Table 9-1 lays out the format of a report that estimates the type of injuries that most likely will lead to a professional liability payout.

The major injuries described in Table 9-1 will account for virtually all of the losses incurred by a hospital. The table can be modified to reflect injuries that are significant to a particular hospital. For the time being, factor out all catastrophic injuries (those that are ten or more times greater in settlement value than the typical case) from the average annual average frequency values. More will be said later on how to attach a value to them under "Determining Coverage Limits."

Step 2

Adjust the frequency averages to reflect significant future changes in the hospital's risk climate. If any of the exposure drivers described in the information gathering section above are expected to increase or decrease

Table 9-1 Injury Summary

Nature of Injury	Annual Average Frequency	Annual Average Payout Per Claim	Projected 1989 Aggregate Losses
Unexplained or unexpected death	1	$100,000	$ 100,000
Paralysis, paraplegia, quadriplegia	.6	250,000	150,000
Spinal cord injury	1	150,000	150,000
Nerve injury or neurologic damage	1	300,000	300,000
Brain damage	1	200,000	200,000
Total or partial loss of a limb or loss of use of a limb	.3	75,000	22,500
Sensory organ or reproductive organ loss or impairment	1	50,000	50,000
Substantial disability or disfigurement	.2	120,000	24,000
Other	.7	10,000	7,000
			$1,003,500

materially, especially in high-risk areas, the frequency estimates should be adjusted accordingly. Material change is defined as a change of 10 percent or more.

Also, if losses have recently been trending upward, the hospital may elect to use the frequency counts from the last several years. A risk manager can stay on top of the hospital's exposures by being involved in a number of administrative processes, including planning, budgeting, and credentialing.

Step 3

Review the accuracy of loss payout estimates. (Losses are defined to include the settlement amount and the costs of investigation and defense for both paid and reserved cases. The hospital should be able to separately identify the amount of each of the two broad payment classifications.) Settlement costs, particularly over the most recent years, have been subject to a great deal of variation. Tort reform changes and spiraling civil justice system award amounts in certain jurisdictions may rule out using institutional historical loss averages in predicting future liability. Hospital staff

Exhibit 9-1 Synopsis of Tort Reform Legislation and Its Potential Impact on Settlements

Collateral Source Rule Changes	This reform provides that the amount of a reward will be reduced by recoveries from collateral sources, such as disability and medical insurance policies. This reform has helped to reduce awards and settlements in states where evidence of collateral payments can be admitted into evidence.
Caps on Non-Economic Damages	These provisions allow for limits to be placed on that part of the award allocated to such intangible things as pain and suffering, loss of consortium, and mental anguish. These caps do not include any portion of the award that relates to out-of-pocket past, present, or future expenses. This reform has helped to make verdicts more predictable and less likely to be influenced by sympathy. In states that have imposed these caps, verdicts have been reduced.
Mandatory Periodic Payments	This reform requires the plaintiff to accept that portion of the award designated as future payments to be accepted in regular installments over a fixed period. (This is most often mandated in cases where future medical expenses represent the bulk of the award.) This reform has not only reduced the overall cost of the settlement and allowed for the defendant to fund the loss over time, but has also helped to guarantee that the injured plaintiff will have money available through his or her lifetime to provide for medical care.
Punitive Damage Award Restrictions	This reform restricts the amount a plaintiff can recover as punitive damages. In some instances, these damages are eliminated entirely or are limited to the most flagrant torts. Although this reform can serve to limit recovery, it can also force juries to include a punitive component in their compensatory damage award.
Immunity Statutes	Such statutes exempt certain individuals, institutions, or public entities from tort liability under specified circumstances or place limits on the amount of recovery a plaintiff may recover from them. A number of these statutes have been successfully challenged on constitutional grounds, thus the protection afforded today by them is questionable.
Frivolous Suit Penalties	Some states have enacted legislation that allows the court to award attorney fees to the opposing party if the suit is found to be groundless. The effect of this provision is that plaintiffs' attorneys must carefully scrutinize facts of a case for the presence of negligence prior to filing a suit or risk having to pay the fees of the opposing party.
Mandatory Pre-Suit Screening or Arbitration	These provisions mandate that prior to the filing of a lawsuit, parties meet before either a panel of peers (from both the medical and legal arenas) and review

Exhibit 9-1 continued

	facts at issue for evidence of negligence or present their case to an arbitration panel that will attempt to assist in early resolution of claims based on facts presented by both parties. Obviously both of these procedures can assist in limiting the number of lawsuits filed. They can also result in a substantial decrease in the costs associated with litigation.
Limitations of Attorneys' Fees	Although many liability suits allow for the awarding of attorneys' fees on a contingency fee basis, this reform provision allows for the court to review and, in some cases, limit the total fee paid to any attorney. This provision obviously can help to reduce the overall damage award.
Expert Witness Laws	These tort reform provisions mandate that persons being called to testify as experts in negligence cases meet certain criteria which qualify them to testify. These criteria might include: current state licensing, board certification in the same specialty as the defendant, training or experience in the same specialty as the defendant—with practice in this area during the year preceding the alleged act of negligence. This will limit the number of "hired gun" experts who are used to testify in cases which are unrelated to their areas of expertise.
Abolition of Joint and Several Liability	This provision limits the ability of the plaintiff to collect an entire amount (or disproportional share of an award) from a defendant who has minimal exposure in a claim. This limits the so-called "deep pocket liability" against the defendant with the greatest assets or largest insurance policy and, rather, apportions damages based on fault.

can review newspaper releases and court records or subscribe to a claims-reporting service such as *Jury Verdict Reporter* to determine the local settlement value of injuries. The services of a skilled trial attorney should also be retained to provide a second opinion as to the estimate of the values developed in connection with Table 9-1. Exhibit 9-1 contains a synopsis of tort reform legislation and its potential impact on settlements. It is important to remember that the true impact of tort reform statutes may not be known until several years after their passage.

DETERMINING COVERAGE LIMITS

The loss frequency and cost data derived from the previous section are a starting point in determining the level of coverage required. Given the nature of professional liability losses (the randomness of events, particularly at a catastrophic level), it is important to determine how often annual losses have exceeded either the historical averages or the estimates reflecting the current court climate. Two loss history compilations are suggested to begin this assessment. Figure 9-1 stratifies past payouts by dollar amount. Figure 9-2 compares the projected losses determined in step 2 to past annual aggregate losses:

Losses can be grouped into these classes:

Level	Description
Baseline	Occur with a predictable frequency and aggregate cost.
Midlevel	Occur in frequency perhaps once every two or three years. Usually are five to ten times higher in settlement value than the baseline average case.
Catastrophic	May never have occurred or can be expected to occur once in a decade or the history of the hospital. Will involve a settlement in the million dollar plus range.

To avoid an unforeseen significant drain on their fiscal resources, hospitals either commercially insure or fund a self-insurance program. Before deciding which coverage option to select, the institution must evaluate the

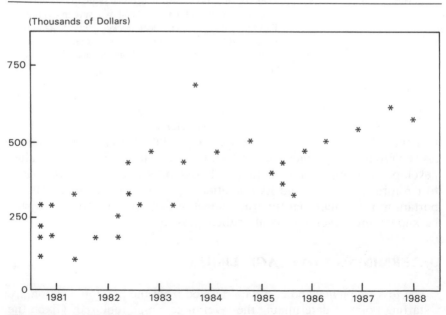

Figure 9-1 Loss Distribution

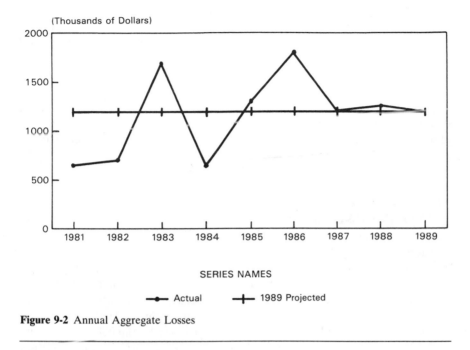

Figure 9-2 Annual Aggregate Losses

---

magnitude of loss exposures it faces. Once potential losses have been quantified, the cost of various forms of coverage can be compared.

Professional liability programs typically insure both individual and aggregate losses. From an aggregate standpoint, at a minimum, hospitals must always commercially insure or self-insure the baseline and at least a portion of the midlevel type of losses. The predicted loss schedule (Table 9-1), modified to reflect current settlement experience, should form the universe of these risks. To the extent that aggregate annual losses historically have frequently exceeded the projected losses, it may be prudent to obtain coverage at least equal to the highest annual past aggregate dollar payout level or the single highest settlement amount. For example, in Figure 9-2 the institution should consider insuring to the aggregate of all actual losses in years 1983 and 1986. Also, if catastrophic settlements have been experienced at other area institutions in clinical programs common to your hospital (even though you may not have had one), it is prudent to insure above the protected payouts on Table 9-1. The risk manager must determine if past above-average losses are an anomaly or can be expected to recur before deciding on how much coverage to have in place.

Individual claim limits are established in conjunction with commercial insurers. Insurance companies often set the per claim limit at a fraction of the aggregate coverage being sought (generally half of the aggregate limit or as a per claim deductible in the midlevel loss range). Given the hospital's loss history or that of the community, the individual loss limit is open to negotiation. If the institution has frequent midlevel losses (several per year) and/or a catastrophic loss every year or so, the individual limit will be set at a relatively high level. On the other hand, hospitals with few midlevel and no catastrophic level losses will be able to seek lower limits.

One last consideration in regard to coverage limits: Often long-term debt issues and vendor contracts stipulate how much coverage must be minimally maintained. Check with your finance officer or purchasing director to determine if such covenants apply.

THE ROLE OF AN ACTUARY IN DETERMINING LIMITS

There are many instances in which the risk manager will need greater precision in the financial and limit analyses than would be available from the historical institutional experience alone. In such instances, it may be appropriate to take advantage of the services of a consulting actuary to take the available loss and exposure information and provide projections of reserves and future losses. This section will describe the role of a casualty actuary and explore some of the applications of actuarial analyses in limit selection, as opposed to the more generalized approach described earlier. It will define the output of such analysis and will attempt to describe the techniques of actuaries.

Perhaps the greatest value of the casualty actuary is the breadth of knowledge and experience that individual brings for projecting losses. For example, some casualty actuaries specialize in projecting the losses of hospitals and other medical facilities. For this reason, the actuary can supplement the hospital's losses with both data from other sources and experienced professional judgment. Other sources of data include the rate filings of insurers in the state, the Insurance Services Office (ISO), and possibly other self-insured institutions. Very often, smaller health care institutions relying exclusively on their own loss data do not have sufficient credibility for either past reserving or for projecting the value of losses into the future. The presence or absence of a single large loss may tremendously influence a loss projection. By melding the experience of other similar institutions into the projections, the projection has more long-term accuracy.

There are at least three instances when a risk manager may wish to employ a casualty actuary to review the loss data. Very often the importance of a decision (e.g., to self-insure or not) may dictate seeking professional advice. In addition, actuaries are called in when there is a merger of two hospitals and there is a need to evaluate current liabilities more accurately.

Finally, the reason may be comparatively straightforward—for example, there are no accurate records of claims or the hospital has substantially altered its risk profile.

An actuarial analysis begins with loss and exposure data from the hospital, such as those listed on the first page of this chapter. The loss data should start with the current values of loss and expense payments and reserves. Ideally, it would also include historical evaluations of these claims, presented at annual intervals.

When the hospital risk manager is evaluating alternative levels of protection for limits, the actuarial analysis can provide an important supporting role. In particular, the actuary can simulate the hospital's losses in the next year to identify the range of potential outcomes. The result of the simulation will be the magnitude of loss at selected confidence intervals. (Simply defined, a confidence interval is a measure of the probability of losses exceeding a certain amount.) This analysis can be used to demonstrate severe (although not necessarily worst case) loss outcomes and the probability that they will occur. The most conservative outcomes of the simulations may be selected as a limit for insurance.

CONCLUSION

The methods used by actuaries represent an alternative or supplement to the method presented in step 3. The information provided by an actuary should also be applied in examining which limits to select. Ultimately, selection should be based on the prudent preservation of the assets of the hospital in the face of adverse loss experience.

chapter 10

Professional Liability Exposures: Self-Insurance Alternatives to Commercial Coverage

Rodney Klein
Tom M. Jones

Over the last decade there has been a greater assumption of professional liability risk on the part of hospitals. The move to self-insurance is the result of the unpredictability of commercial insurance, both in terms of price and availability. Self-insurance, in the case of smaller hospitals, usually involves a loss deductible in the range of $25,000 to $100,000. On the other end of the spectrum, larger and more clinically complicated institutions can retain millions of dollars of first-dollar risk, replacing the need to purchase primary insurance coverage. The vast majority of hospitals with over 250 beds in high-risk jurisdictions are in the latter category.

The principal reasons for self-insuring are relatively straightforward. Insurers generally no longer offer first-dollar coverage, and if it is available, it is prohibitively expensive. Also, self-insuring substantially influences the cost of buying insurance. Other benefits result from self-insuring:

- Improved loss prevention: Once an institution becomes responsible for payment of its own loss, there is more motivation to emphasize sound loss prevention programs that will potentially reduce exposure.
- Improved claims control: The self-insured maintain greater control over claims. That includes control over the accumulation of loss and exposure data and data concerning the disposition of claims and suits, control over the quality of the defense and investigation of a claim,

and control over the amount of reserves maintained for payment of claims.

- Improved cost control: Less overhead is associated with claims handling and administration; the self-insured avoids commissions, profits, premium taxes, and other fronting costs. Such costs are a substantial part of every premium dollar paid.
- Cash flow benefits: Loss reserves are controlled by the self-insured, giving them an opportunity to invest their funds in a more profitable manner.

To the extent that the insured does not adequately fund or administer the risks being assumed, the results can be fiscally devastating.

This chapter will concentrate on three topics:

1. determining the optimal amount of commercial insurance to obtain versus self-insuring
2. determining the amount of funds that must be set aside to meet self-insurance obligations
3. exploring various legal structures available to control the investment of self-insurance funding and to facilitate the purchase of coverage in excess of self-insurance limits

HOW MUCH TO SELF-INSURE

A three-step process is recommended to arrive at a reasonable estimate on how much to self-insure.

Step 1

Recall the discussion in Chapter 9 relative to the three strata of losses: baseline, midlevel, and catastrophic. Predictable losses (baseline and, to a certain extent, a portion of the midlevel losses) should be self-insured. An insurer will examine your past loss history and include the cost of these losses dollar for dollar in its premium. In addition to the insurer's out-of-pocket costs, the premium will contain a markup for underwriting profits, brokers' commissions, and various taxes. The current insurance policy may also cover claims investigation and defense costs that may be transferred to the hospital under a self-insurance program. If you are going to insure these costs in any event, why pay the markup? As midlevel losses potentially do not occur every year, an average value of this class of loss could be self-insured.

If a hospital has a possible ongoing exposure to catastrophic losses, it should not self-insure such losses. The fiscal resources of the health care industry are declining, making it highly unlikely an institution could weather a catastrophic loss, especially more than once over a several-year period.

The following list contains the attributes that determine the ability of a hospital to retain risk:

1. fiscal strength
2. quality of internal risk management processes
3. quality and cooperativeness of the medical staff
4. volume of high-risk clinical services being provided
5. settlement climate in its market area
6. competence of trial counsel
7. effectiveness of state tort reform statutes
8. past loss history of the institution and its perception in the community
9. type of patients seen

Of all of the attributes, the effectiveness of the risk management and quality assurance programs has the most significant bearing on the hospital's professional liability exposure.

The insurer also has a say in how much risk the institution must bear. Minimum retentions vary by company and the complexity of the hospital's operations. Professional liability insurance is a seller's market.

Step 2

Seek alternate insurance price quotations. It is important to test the premium savings that can be achieved at various levels of self-insurance. The overhead markup included in the cost of insurance often exceeds 25 percent. The "savings" in premium becomes the collateral to pay for the risk being retained.

Self-insurance proposals can be crafted in several ways:

- The hospital can set its risk retention at some portion of its expected per case and aggregate losses, ranging from the base level into the catastrophic layer.
- The institution's broker, knowing the insurance marketplace, can propose retentions that make sense.

- Underwriters may dictate, given the size and complexity of the hospital, what retention levels are minimally acceptable.

Step 3

Test the reasonableness of the savings in premium to be achieved by self-insuring. In order to perform the test, it is essential to determine, based on historical losses, the insurer's risk exposure on an individual claims basis and in the aggregate. The analysis technique that follows assumes (1) adoption of a self-insurance retention of $500,000 per occurrence and $2,000,000 in the aggregate (with the hospital currently carrying first-dollar coverage of $5,500,000 per occurrence and $7,000,000 in the aggregate) and (2) purchase of excess insurance of $5,000,000 per occurrence and $5,000,000 in the aggregate, above the self-retention.

The data arranged in Figures 10-1 and 10-2 can represent loss history on a claims made or occurrence basis to properly match the form of commercial insurance coverage being purchased.

Per Occurrence Analysis

Compile the value of historical losses above the occurrence retention limit. The historical losses must be inflated to reflect the inflationary trend in individual settlement values, which range from 15 to 25 percent. This will allow the hospital to quantify the risks the insurer is no longer facing

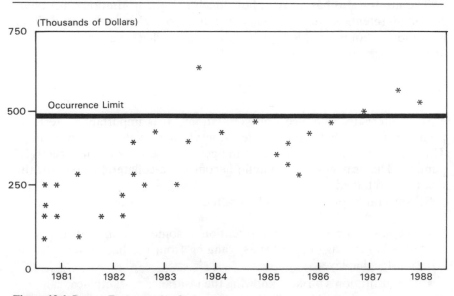

Figure 10-1 Payout Frequency by Occurrence

and, conversely, the risks the insurer remains exposed to. (See Figure 10-1.)

Aggregate Analysis

Compile the aggregate of all historical inflated losses. (See Figure 10-2.)

Determining the Reasonableness of the Insurer's Quote

The best test of an insurer's price quotation, when contemplating a significant self-assumption of risk, is to discount the prior year's premium quotation by the estimated risk being borne by the hospital. By comparing this calculation to the quote for next year, provided by the insurer, the quote should be no more than 20 percent above your calculated value (again, the 20 percent represents various fees, commissions, and inflation).

The second test of reasonableness quantifies the dollar value of exposures per occurrence and in the aggregate that faces the insurer. (See Table 10-1.) Again, the historical losses have been adjusted for inflation.

From the insurer's standpoint in Table 10-1, given the concentration of losses above the retention limits in recent years, a premium in the $100,000 to $200,000 range would not be inappropriate for the risk being assumed

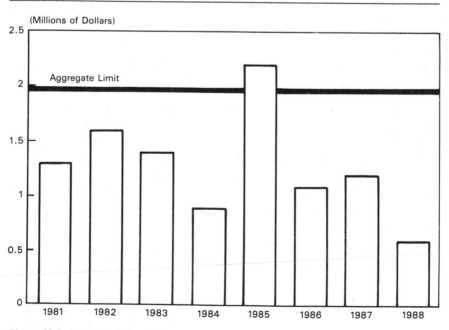

Figure 10-2 Aggregate Payout Summary

Table 10-1 Losses Exceeding Self-Insured Retention

	Per Occurrence	Aggregate	Total
1981			
1982			
1983	$100,000		$100,000
1984			
1985		$200,000	200,000
1986	50,000		50,000
1987	100,000		100,000
1988	75,000		75,000
TOTAL	$325,000	$200,000	$525,000
AVERAGE			$ 65,625

by the insurer. As explained previously, factors other than the hospital's loss history may have a bearing on the premium charged by the insurer:

- recent catastrophic losses in the hospital's market in clinical programs common to the insured
- expansion or contraction of high-risk services
- minimum pricing standards of the insurer. (Certain companies have a minimum premium that is charged to the best of risks, regardless of whether their losses are substantially below the premium.)
- tort reform amendments
- the provision of support services in regard to loss reporting, claims defense, and settlement

If the hospital is converting its coverage from an occurrence to a claims made basis, the premium from the prior year will be relatively higher. A claims made policy, given the time span it takes to report all compensable events, will result in less liability for the insurer in the first three to five policy years than an occurrence policy. After about five years, a claims made policy with a retroactive inception date will approximate the premium of an occurrence policy. A claims made policy matures in cost in roughly the following manner:

	Claims-Made Premium as a Percent of an Occurrence Policy
Year 1	40%
Year 2	60%
Year 3	80%
Year 4	90%
Year 5	100%

To the extent that the premiums being quoted are not justified, given the hospital's loss history and the other variables affecting pricing, the broker should attempt to negotiate a fairer price with the insurer.

SELF-INSURANCE FUNDING ANALYSIS

When a hospital is considering entering into a self-insurance program, the decision may dictate the use of actuarial analysis both before and after the decision. Before the decision is made, the analysis will provide supporting documentation for decision-making purposes. If a program is implemented, then an annual actuarial analysis should be conducted to define the proper level of funding for the program.

When a hospital is examining self-insurance, an actuarial analysis provides important information to assist in decision making. As described previously, the self-insurance evaluation needs to take into account the expected loss that would be assumed and losses that would be transferred under the scenario. This would include estimates of loss adjustment expenses that are characteristic of the geographic area and financing alternatives. This is the primary result of such an analysis.

Related to this, a second result of the analysis should be the expected losses under alternative levels of self-insured retention. For example, the hospital risk manager may be presented with a series of risk financing alternatives involving different levels of self-insured retention. While in some cases the health care institution may not have experienced a loss with a given level of retention, that does not exclude the possibility that such a loss may occur in the future. By taking advantage of a broader database of information, the actuary is able to provide a reasonable estimate of the possibility of loss within that particular level of retention.

The actuarial analysis should also present information related to the potential for adverse deviation within a given retention. For example, the analysis may indicate that while losses are expected to be $2,000,000 within a $100,000 specific retention, there is a 20 percent chance they will exceed $2,800,000. These scenarios may also be contemplated in such an analysis. This information can be used to test the hospital's economic and psychological appetite for accepting greater swings in year-to-year cost.

When a self-insurance program has been established for financing, the hospital is generally required by Medicare and its creditors to conduct an annual analysis of the reserves that would be needed to fund the trust fund. This analysis can provide reserves at selected confidence intervals.

Finally, in the application of a self-insurance program internally, many hospitals have begun to allocate the costs of insurance and self-insurance funding to the various departments. The actuary can provide an allocation technique that reflects both the inherent exposure of the procedures that are conducted within the department and some measure of the fluctuation of the losses that have occurred within that department over the past. The blend between the exposure of the department and its experience is best determined based upon objective factors such as the size and years of loss experience (credibility) of the department and subjective factors such as the content of the hospital's risk control program.

One issue that must continuously be examined once a self-insurance program is implemented is that of the level of funding. A broad spectrum of funding approaches is available, ranging from "pay-as-you-go" to fully funded with a conservative reserve margin. A pay-as-you-go approach relies on an estimate of actual cash outlays for the forthcoming year. Clearly, this represents the least allocation of resources, but it delays recognition of actual liabilities incurred. A second approach is to fund for the value of claims made during the course of the year. That is more conservative and corresponds to an occurrence-based excess insurance program. The first approach delays recognition of unreported liabilities incurred in a year. The most conservative approach is to fund for all potential uninsured losses occurring in a year, including a margin for adverse loss experience. This approach, which involves the greatest up-front cost, clearly recognizes all liabilities. The actual funding technique selected should be based on the financial capabilities of the hospital, the dictates of financial management, and the requirements of auditors.

An important consideration in establishing and operating a self-insurance program is that the program should not be evaluated based on the results of a single year of operation. While the actuarial analysis will suggest alternative levels of funding, the year-to-year losses may deviate, perhaps substantially, from these amounts. For that reason, the financial and risk management benefits of the self-insurance program should be re-examined over a period of five or more years.

LEGAL STRUCTURES

A number of factors necessitate that a legal structure apart from the hospital itself be established to handle the affairs of a self-insurance program. Medicare reimbursement guidelines remain the key reason. Other factors include the ability to protect the self-insurance assets from being used to satisfy other obligations, using the legal structure to expand the brokerage role played by the insured(s), and allowing the insured(s) to create hybrid insurance products.

The following section will focus on the general Medicare requirements governing self-insured programs. Then, the advantages and disadvantages of various alternative legal structures will be briefly reviewed.

General Medicare Guidelines

Basic Requirements

Payments made to a self-insurance trust fund established to finance the professional liability risks of a single entity or of a group or pool will be reimbursable under the Medicare program if the program's requirements are satisfied. Self-insurance is defined by Medicare as "a means whereby a provider(s), whether proprietary or nonproprietary, undertakes the risk to protect itself against anticipated liabilities by providing funds in an amount equivalent to liquidate those liabilities." If there is any shifting of risk to an unrelated party, the arrangement will not be treated as self-insurance for reimbursement purposes but simply as a commercial insurance expense.

Establishing a Trust Fund

Medicare requires that each self-insured provider or the self-insurance pool establish "a fund with a recognized independent fiduciary such as a bank, a trust company, or a private benefit administrator." The provider or pool must also enter into a written agreement with the fiduciary, containing all of the following provisions. First, the agreement must include all appropriate legal responsibilities and obligations of the fiduciary as required by state laws. Second, the fiduciary must have legal title to the trust fund and be responsible for its proper administration and control. Third, the fiduciary may not be related to the provider either through ownership or control, unless the fiduciary is a state acting on the behalf of a state or local governmental provider or pool. In this regard, the fiduciary's power to make investments shall be limited to those approved under state law governing the use of such fund; however, the fiduciary may not make any loans from the fund to the provider or persons related to the provider.

Fiduciary Agreement

The fiduciary agreement must also provide that withdrawals may be made only for malpractice and comprehensive general liability, losses, or administration expenses reimbursable by Medicare. If it is established that there is a practice of making payments from the fund for purposes unrelated to its proper administration, this "may result in a withdrawal of recognition of the self-insurance fund by the Medicare program. In such instances, payments into the fund will not be considered an allowable cost."

The fiduciary agreement must provide for any income earned by the fund to become part of the fund and to be used in establishing adequate fund levels.

Medicare also requires an annual certified statement from an independent actuary, insurance company, or broker with actuarial personnel experienced in medical malpractice and general liability insurance; the agent must be independent from the provider in terms of direct or indirect financial ownership or control. This statement must contain a determination of the amount necessary to pay into the fund in order to provide "reserves for losses based on accepted actuarial techniques customarily employed by the section of the insurance industry writing the type of insurance coverage the fund is designed to provide, and expenses relating to the self-insurance trust fund," which are reimbursable under the Medicare program. The statement must also contain an estimate of any amounts of the fund in excess of what is reasonably required to support anticipated disbursements from the fund. Such excess contributions will not be allowable costs for the period in question, but they may be allowed in a subsequent reporting period.

The actuary, insurance company, or broker making the annual certified statement must describe the actuarial basis and coverage period used in establishing reserve levels. Reserves will not be recognized, however, as allowable costs under the Medicare program for losses specifically denied by Medicare regulations. Payments to establish reserves will not be recognized for items such as (1) losses in excess of the greater of 10 percent of a provider's net worth or $100,000, where a provider elects to pay losses directly in lieu of establishing a funded self-insurance fund, or (2) losses in excess of coverage levels that Medicare deems do not reflect the decisions of prudent management.

Risk Management and Claims Administration

A self-insured provider or pool must also satisfy Medicare that it has an ongoing claims process, and claims adjustment services may be provided either by the qualified personnel of a provider or pool or by an independent contractor such as an insurance company. The self-insured provider or pool is also required to obtain adequate legal assistance for carrying out its claims process. In addition, each self-insured provider must have an adequate risk management program. The mandatory risk management program must have the same characteristics as programs required by commercial insurers for the same risks. A self-insured provider must therefore maintain an ongoing safety program, a professional and employee training program, and other programs necessary to minimize the frequency and severity of malpractice and comprehensive general liability incidents.

Reimbursable Expenses of Administration

Medicare provides that only the following expenses will be treated as costs attributable to a single entity or pooled self-insurance trust fund:

> expenses of establishing the provider fund or pool, expenses for administering the claims management program, expenses involved with maintenance of the fund by the fiduciary, legal expenses, actuarial expenses, excess insurance coverage (if purchased by the fiduciary or pool), risk management (if performed by the fiduciary or pool), and a coordination of benefits program (if performed by the fiduciary, pool, or provider) to the extent that such expenses are related to the provider's self-insurance program.

All other expenses will not be treated as costs attributable to the self-insurance trust fund.

Alternative Legal Structures for Self-Insurance

Background

In addition to or in lieu of a self-insured retention (often in the trust format described above), various more complex structures are being used by hospitals as risk retention devices. These structures typically take the form of liability insurance risk purchasing groups, risk retention groups, or offshore captive insurance companies. While the suitability of each format to a particular situation, as well as its particular advantages and disadvantages, varies widely, certain common threads run through all these self-insurance vehicles.

First, they are most applicable to multihospital or combined hospital/nonemployed physician programs. A single hospital usually is best off with a simple trust. The remainder of this discussion will be limited to liability coverage of the hospital and its employed physicians or allied health professionals. (Under the legal doctrine of *respondeat superior*, an employer is automatically responsible for the errors and omissions of employees if made within the scope of employment.) So-called channeled insurance programs in which hospitals sponsor professional liability insurance for selected independent contractor physicians, a substantial portion of whose practice is at a sponsoring hospital, is an extremely complex subject not addressed here.

Second, these exotic formats invariably are more expensive and time-consuming than trusts to implement and operate. In addition to increased legal fees arising out of state insurance regulatory compliance and possible securities law registration or disclosure, multihospital insurers generally are subject to federal income tax regardless of their form. Moreover, multi-owner governance and control issues dictate a carefully planned set of bylaws and a shareholders' stock buy-back agreement. Having made the foregoing warnings, a brief description of these alternatives, with their basic pros and cons, follows.

Purchasing Groups

If a commercial carrier desirous of insuring the multiowner group can be found, the easiest approach is an insurance "purchasing group" formed pursuant to facilitating provisions of the Liability Risk Retention Act of 1986. This federal statute provides a limited pre-emption of state "anti-fictitious group" insurance laws, thus permitting a single carrier to issue a group policy to hospitals in various jurisdictions. Unfortunately, the courts have strictly construed this federal pre-emption, such that state laws re-quiring the insurer to be admitted or otherwise approved by the insurance department of every state where an insured hospital purchasing group member is located have been upheld. In addition, state laws mandating that policy terms and premium rates be filed and in some cases preapproved have been held valid. Accordingly, the usefulness of purchasing groups, at least in a multijurisdictional context, is in doubt.

Retained Risk Arrangements

Unlike purchasing groups, which retain no risk and therefore require no capitalization, both offshore "captives" and domestic risk retention groups (RRGs) in essence are privately owned insurance companies subject to statutory and actuarial capital and surplus requirements. A key objective of forming an offshore captive or RRG is to achieve some measure of stability in the historically volatile medical malpractice liability insurance area by using this capital as a "buffer" to smooth excessive fluctuations in premium rates. A purchasing group that is totally reliant on a commercial carrier subject to the industry's cyclical insurance swings is of little use to enhance coverage availability and pricing consistency. A few common fea-tures of both the offshore captive and RRG forms of self-insurance will be mentioned, then their major distinguishing characteristics will be outlined.

Both offshore captives and RRGs typically provide an intermediate level of funded self-insurance that provides coverage over a self-insured retention and under excess liability insurance obtained in the commercial markets. Often, but not always, a substantial portion of the captive's or RRG's retained risk will be commercially reinsured either in United States or London markets. The actuarial determination of the appropriate capitalization and premium is identical for both formats, although differences in taxation, briefly discussed below, should be taken into account.

Operational aspects and financial rules of thumb are similar for both offshore captives and RRGs. For example, both usually are managed in the chartering jurisdiction by contract with a third party service provider, which also may provide claims administration and risk management services to the captive or RRG. Traditional insurance ratios are applied to both by regulators when deciding whether to grant a license to transact an insurance business. For example, one such ratio indicates that generally premiums should not exceed three times capital and surplus. Another is that capital should be at least five to ten times exposure to any single risk. A chart showing the minimum capital requirements and other characteristics of popular offshore captive and RRG chartering jurisdictions can be found in Table 10-2.

Offshore Captives. Originally developed by multinational corporations largely as a means of tax savings, offshore captives have evolved over the past 20 years into a highly developed industry. The most popular chartering jurisdictions are tax havens such as the Cayman Islands, Bermuda, Barbados, and the Bahamas. A key element of "going offshore" for tax-exempt hospitals is the opportunity (no longer available to taxable business corporations), with careful structuring and proper tax planning advice, to indefinitely defer United States income tax on their underwriting and investment income. Most captives must pay in lieu of income tax a federal excise tax of 4 percent of gross premiums. Exceptions exist for single parent/insured captives, for captives subject to United States income tax, and for captives formed in Barbados or Bermuda (by treaty exemption expiring on January 1, 1990). If the captive is a reinsurer, then the domestic, unrelated "fronting" company pays only a 1 percent federal excise tax (subject to the foregoing exceptions).

Risk Retention Groups. A fairly recent innovation, RRGs are formed pursuant to a federal statute, the Liability Risk Retention Act of 1986. Various states have enacted facilitating legislation attractive to RRGs. Most popular sites for hospitals that have established RRGs are Vermont, Tennessee, and Colorado. Basically, an RRG can meet the regulatory chartering requirements of any state and by virtue of this federal statute operate

Table 10-2 Comparison of Captive Statutes of Selected Domestic and Offshore Jurisdictions

Types of Captive	Vermont	Tennessee	Bermuda	Cayman Islands
Types of Captive	Pure association, industrial insured (includes risk retention groups)	Pure association, mutual	No special captive legislation	No special captive legislation. Most captives obtain unrestricted Class B insurer's licenses.
Statutory minimum capital and surplus	Pure—$250,000 Association—$750,000 Industrial insured—$500,000	Pure—$750,000 Association/mutual—$1,000,000 ($750,000 if all members are not-for-profit)	General—$120,000 Long-term (e.g., life)—$250,000	General—$120,000 Long-term—$240,000
Letters of credit allowed	Yes	Yes for stock companies; No for mutual captives, unless all members are not-for-profit	Yes—with permission; and only for amounts over minimum capital requirements	Discretionary
Minimum premium	None	Pure: $500,000 Association: $1,000,000 ($500,000 if all members are not-for-profit)	None	None
Investment restrictions	Association: Must comply with investment requirements for domestic insurance companies Rest: None	Investment requirements for stock casualty companies apply; pure captives may obtain exceptions	None	None

	Vermont	Tennessee	Bermuda	Cayman Islands
Office and records	Principal office, books, and records in Vermont	Principal office, books, and records in Tennessee	Principal office, books, and records in Bermuda	Principal office, books, and records in Cayman Islands
Directors and officers	One director must be a Vermont resident	No residency requirements	Two directors must be Bermuda residents	No residency requirements
Rates and forms	No approval required	May require filing of forms; rates may not be excessive, inadequate, or unfairly discriminatory	No approval required	No approval required
Reserve/underwriting requirements	Actuarial opinion on reserves required annually	Regulators want to see some Tennessee risks	Statutory capital and surplus must be at least $120,000 for net premium income (NPI) up to $600,000; 20% of NPI for NPI of $600,000 to $6 million; and 10% of NPI plus $600,000 for NPI over $6 million	Generally, surplus should not be less than 1/5 of annual premiums
Reporting requirements	Annual GAAP financial statement; convention statement for association captives	Annual convention statement	Annual statutory financial return	Auditor's certificate and "certificate of compliance"

in the other 49 states with only minimal regulation. Thus, an RRG is ideally suited for a multistate affiliation of hospitals where an offshore captive is inappropriate because, for example, sufficient onshore activity will occur to risk violation of the states' prohibition of transacting an insurance business in the particular state without a license. Unlike a carefully structured and operated offshore captive, an RRG is automatically subject to federal income tax on its underwriting and investment income. This disadvantage disappears, however, if the offshore captive purposely or inadvertently engages in a United States trade or business, or if its shareholders are taxable entities. A final requirement to qualify as an RRG is that every owner be an insured and every insured be an owner. This egalitarian approach sometimes leads to questions of corporate governance and control since the legislative history evidences a distaste for entrepreneurial uses of this statute.

chapter 11

An Overview of the Insurance Marketplace

Catherine T. Hartlieb

The hospital professional liability insurance marketplace opened the door to the hard insurance market in both the 1970s and the 1980s and never really closed that door. Recovery from each hard market encounter has left a dramatic and indelible mark on the financial profile of the hospital industry and has created a need for individual hospitals to develop an active risk management program to protect their balance sheets.

In the 1970s the hard market drastically reduced the limits available, substantially increased the premiums, and forced large hospitals or those in high-risk jurisdictions to self-insure the first $1 million per occurrence, with annual aggregates of $3 million. In reality, this means that hospitals now self-insure the primary layer for professional liability. Because of this, hospitals were forced to become familiar with the basic elements of an insurance company: funding, risk management, claims management, and defense selection. They were also forced to develop new programs and hire additional staff to perform these new functions.

In the 1980s the hard market even more harshly duplicated the 1970s, resulting in the addition of two new components:

(1) Claims made coverage replaced traditional "occurrence" coverage in most markets for those seeking individual facultative reinsurance placement, and
(2) Increased self-insurance became mandatory. Hospitals were forced to self-insure more and to purchase additional excess coverage. Many also became involved in excess pooling arrangements with other hospitals.

In the autumn and winter of 1988, the hospital professional liability insurance marketplace stabilized. Limit capacity is readily available, premium ranges vary from 10 percent reductions to a 10 percent increase, and

151

there is a slight element of competitiveness between companies offering the product. Table 11-1 identifies the dominant companies providing primary and excess hospital professional liability coverage (both domestic and foreign), cites their coverages and liability limits, and gives the Best's ratings for domestic insurers. The latter are taken from *Best's Insurance*

Table 11-1 Hospital Professional Liability Overview

	Coverage	Total Limit*	Best's Rating
Domestic Primary and Excess Companies			
St. Paul	CM,Ded/SIR	$40,000,000**	A XI
Continental	CM,Ded/SIR	11,000,000	A XIII
National Union-Lexington	CM,Ded/SIR	16,000,000	A+ XIV
PHICO	CM,Ded/SIR	11,000,000	B+ VII
ACIC (MMI)	CM,Ded/SIR (occurrence buffer)	11,000,000 1,000,000	B VI
Virginia Insurance Reciprocal	CM,Ded/SIR	9,000,000	A V
Farmers Insurance Group	Modified occurrence	40,000,000***	A+ XIV
Travelers	CM,Ded/SIR	27,500,000	A XV
AIG Risk Management	Fronting only		A+ XIV
Domestic Excess Companies			
Employers Reinsurance Corp. (A+X)	CM or Occurrence Reinsurance only	25,000,000	See individual fronting co.
Hospital Providers Insurance Co. (HPIC)	CM or Occurrence	Quota share 2,500,000	None (American Hospital Association owned)
	Claims Made only	5,000,000 excess of 6,000,000	
Bershire Hathaway	CM or Occurrence	5,000,000 in-house	A+ X
(Columbia)	ERC Front	25,000,000	
Reliance Insurance Cos.	CM or Occurrence	5,000,000 in-house	A VII
	ERC Front	25,000,000	
Foreign Excess Companies			
Weavers	CM	$ 5,000,000 (Plus % of top layers)	NA
Lexington (London)	CM	10,000,000	
Merrett (Lloyds)	CM	Quota Share	NA
Turegum (Zurich)	CM	Quota Share	NA
Union America (Continental)	CM	Quota Share	NA

*The capacity of any company is subject to change depending on reinsurance market conditions.
**Includes $25,000,000 Employers Reinsurance Corp. participation.
***Total state program capacity, including the European market, exclusive of Employers Reinsurance Corp. participation.

Table 11-1 (continued)

Coverage	Total Limit*	Best's Rating
CNA Reinsurance (London)	CM	Quota Share	A + XV
Hanover Reinsurance (London)	CM	Quota Share	

*The capacity of any company is subject to change depending on reinsurance market conditions.

Note:

CM, claims made coverage
Ded/SIR, deductible or self-insured retention
Occurrence Buffer, the amount of the loss retained by the insured per each individual loss
Modified Occurrence, type of reporting method that expands strict claims made coverage for the excess layers by allowing for extended reporting

Fronting Only, the company retains no risk
Quota Share, do not take a full line of coverage but rather participate only with other companies on a percentage
ERC Front, Employers Reinsurance Company

Reports—Property and Casualty, which monitors domestic companies' overall performance (by a letter designation, explained in Exhibit 11-1) and financial stability (by a roman numeral designation, explained in Table 11-2).

There is virtually no first-dollar hospital professional liability coverage, and that which is available is very costly. Even the small hospital now maintains a minimum deductible of $25,000 or a self-insured retention (SIR) of $100,000 to $300,000.

SELECTING AN INSURANCE COMPANY

The qualifications in selecting an insurance company are the same for both primary and excess layers. You must select a company that will best serve your individual needs. The following are guides to assist you in this choice.

Financial Stability

An excellent indicator of the industry performance and financial worth of a domestic company is Best's rating, which should be evaluated carefully by your management. Learn as much as you can about the insurance company's history and performance in the health care field.

Exhibit 11-1 Best's Rating Classifications

A + (Superior)

Assigned to those companies which in our opinion have achieved superior overall performance when compared to the norms of the property/casualty insurance industry. A + (Superior) rated insurers generally have demonstrated the strongest ability to meet their respective policyholder and other contractual obligations.

A and A − (Excellent)

Assigned to those companies which in our opinion have achieved excellent overall performance when compared to the norms of the property/casualty insurance industry. A and A − (Excellent) rated insurers generally have demonstrated a strong ability to meet their respective policyholder and other contractual obligations.

B + (Very Good)

Assigned to those companies which in our opinion have achieved very good overall performance when compared to the norms of the property/casualty insurance industry. B + (Very Good) rated insurers generally have demonstrated a very good ability to meet their policyholder and other contractual obligations.

B and B − (Good)

Assigned to those companies which in our opinion have achieved good overall performance when compared to the norms of the property/casualty insurance industry. B and B − (Good) rated insurers generally have demonstrated a good ability to meet their policyholder and other contractual obligations.

C + (Fairly Good)

Assigned to those companies which in our opinion have achieved fairly good overall performance when compared to the norms of the property/casualty insurance industry. C + (Fairly Good) rated insurers generally have demonstrated a fairly good ability to meet their respective policyholder and other contractual obligations.

C and C − (Fair)

Assigned to those companies which in our opinion have achieved fair overall performance when compared to the norms of the property/casualty insurance industry. C and C − (Fair) rated insurers generally have demonstrated a fair ability to meet their policyholder and other contractual obligations.

Table 11-2 Best's Financial Size Category

Financial Size Category		Adjusted Policyholders' Surplus (*thousands of dollars*)
Class I	Up to	1,000
Class II	1,000 to	2,000
Class III	2,000 to	5,000
Class IV	5,000 to	10,000
Class V	10,000 to	25,000
Class VI	25,000 to	50,000
Class VII	50,000 to	100,000
Class VIII	100,000 to	250,000
Class IX	250,000 to	500,000
Class X	500,000 to	750,000
Class XI	750,000 to	1,000,000
Class XII	1,000,000 to	1,250,000
Class XIII	1,250,000 to	1,500,000
Class XIV	1,500,000 to	2,000,000
Class XV	2,000,000 or	more

The *Best's Insurance Reports—Property and Casualty* monitors both the overall performance of the company by the letter designation and the company's financial stability by the roman numeral classification cited above.

Long-Term Commitment

Your insurance company should have a track record of continuing to write coverage through both hard and soft markets. The insurer may have reduced limits and changed from occurrence to claims made coverage, but it should have maintained a line of hospital professional liability coverage during the hard market period. The company must demonstrate commitment to the health care industry. This is a two-way street. The hospital must also endeavor to maintain a long-term commitment to its insurers. Switching insurers each year is very dangerous, especially if claims made coverage is purchased.

Flexible Underwriting Standards

The insurance company underwriters must personally evaluate census statistics and loss data. Computer-driven rating tends to escalate premium costs. The "hands-on" underwriting component is essential to ascertain the most competitive price level. It is recommended that hospital management *personally* meet the underwriter before the renewal terms are formalized.

SELECTING A BROKER

Another important selection is whom you choose to broker your account. There are many insurance brokers, but the leading national health care brokers specialize in hospital professional liability and will save your hospital much in excess premiums and claims payments. The leading national health care brokers are

- Alexander and Alexander
- Carroon and Black
- Frank B. Hall
- Fred S. James
- Johnson and Higgins
- March and McLennan

Broker Responsibilities

Your broker must perform a dual role as your broker and your hospital professional liability consultant. Look for the following attributes in selecting an appropriate broker for your account:

1. personally knows the hospital professional liability insurance market and its leading underwriters
2. understands and is able to explain your coverage
3. is able to keep you advised of any and all hospital professional liability coverage and market changes
4. possesses the respect of your lead underwriter
5. is aggressive in obtaining premium reductions and in constantly updating your program with worthwhile changes
6. is able to design and redesign your hospital professional liability as the market changes from hard to soft or from soft to hard
7. has an in-house risk management staff to augment and complement yours as required
8. has the personnel and ability to properly report claims, especially if claims coverage is purchased
9. can assist you in producing a loss run that correctly lists your claims, in a format that is acceptable to the underwriter

10. purchases professional errors and omissions coverage and gives you certification
11. offers to work on either a straight commission or fee basis. (Ask up-front what percentage of a commission is earned for the placement of insurance. If additional consultant or referral fees are also charged, they should be discussed up-front.)

Hospital Responsibilities

To maximize the benefits of the broker/hospital relationship, the hospital must also accept certain responsibilities. Among these responsibilities are the following:

- The hospital must declare and explain all of the operations and risk exposures at policy inception each year.
- The hospital should immediately advise the broker (consultant) about any changes or additions to the declared operation during the policy period.
- The hospital must endorse active risk management.
- The hospital must produce accurate loss runs each quarter, which delineate paid losses, expenses and indemnity, reserved losses, and an evaluation of incurred but not reported losses.
- The hospital must take the time to *read* its hospital professional liability policies and *understand* the terms and obligations.
- The hospital must obtain written clarification of gray areas in policies from either the insurer or the broker (consultant)

chapter 12

Understanding Policy Terms and Features

Michael D. Sheppard

As a hospital risk manager, one must develop a working knowledge and understanding of the insurance policies purchased for the organization.

Most insurance policies today are written in easy-to-read language for the policyholder. (Some policies, such as the Lloyds of London forms, contain more complex language.) However, an understanding of basic policy format will diminish any confusion that may arise at the time of a loss. The risk manager must learn how to apply the policy language to the everyday exposures the hospital faces. Too often, insurance policy language is ignored until there is a dispute with the carrier or a denial of coverage for a claim. A good risk manager will understand the applicability of the policy to situations as they occur.

When a policy is issued or renewed, one should review it in detail to be certain that the policy terminology reflects exactly the coverage sought. Any discrepancies should be immediately brought to the attention of the broker and the underwriter. Additionally, it is often helpful to review the policy language at the time an incident occurs to make certain that the proper coverage exists.

COMMON TYPES OF INSURANCE FOR HOSPITALS

The predominant exposure for the hospital or health care environment is that of professional liability. At least two liability policies are needed when there is a professional liability exposure; (1) *professional liability insurance,* which provides coverage for liability arising from rendering of or failure to render professional services; (2) *general liability insurance,* which provides coverage for liability arising out of the hazards of a hospital's premises and operations.

The most common form of insurance secured by hospitals is the hospital professional liability (HPL) policy. This form protects the hospital against claims for injury arising out of a medical incident.

The comprehensive general liability (CGL) policy protects the hospital against claims for injury or damage that occurs on the premises or arises out of the more concrete operations of the hospital.

There are four distinctions between these two policies:

1. The HPL form usually contains a single insuring clause and restricts the coverage to bodily injury; the CGL form provides coverage for bodily injury and property damage.
2. The HPL form covers damages arising out of the rendering of professional services and is not intended to substitute for public liability coverage.
3. The injury covered in the HPL form is not restricted to being caused by an accident or occurrence, as it is in the CGL form.
4. The HPL form usually requires the formal consent of the policyholder prior to the settlement of any claim made under the policy; consent to settlement is not available under CGL coverage.

Most hospital insurers today underwrite both professional liability coverage and premises and operations coverage under the HPL form to avoid disputes over the applicability of coverage in certain situations (e.g., patient injuries and/or deaths as a result of a hospital fire).

The structure of the coverage can vary from carrier to carrier to meet the needs and requirements of the individual hospital risk. Many carriers offer self-insured retentions or deductibles wherein the insured hospital retains the first level of monetary exposure for claims under the policy. The dollar amount of this retention is negotiable with the underwriter and is based on the risk and financial status of the individual hospital.

Nonmedical professional liability insurance is commonly referred to as *errors and omissions coverage* (E & O). The coverage is basically the same except that bodily injury is usually excluded on these forms. A good example of a profession that requires E & O coverage is accountancy. Accountants hold themselves out to the public as possessing certain skills and expertise in their field. When a mistake or an error is made by an accountant, resulting in damage to others, the need arises for professional liability protection. E & O policies are usually tailored to meet the needs of the individual profession they are insuring.

There are always liability exposures above the limits available for all other policies. The *umbrella policy* provides the high limits needed for catastrophic losses, as well as broader coverage than most other liability policies. An umbrella policy serves four basic functions:

1. It raises the limits of the underlying policies to cover catastrophic losses.
2. It normally has broader coverage than the combined scope of the underlying policies.
3. When underlying policy limits are exhausted because of aggregates, or when there is no underlying coverage, the umbrella becomes the primary insurance for defense and related expenses, as well as indemnity for injuries.
4. It covers hazards not insured under other liability policies, such as liability for invasion of privacy in an advertisement or non-owned aircraft liability.

CLAIMS MADE VERSUS OCCURRENCE

Nearly all malpractice and professional liability policies today are written on a claims made basis. This means that if a claim is made against the hospital by a patient, it must be made during the policy period.

The policy does not require the medical incident or malpractice to fall necessarily within the policy period, but the notice of claim must be made during the policy period. For example, a nursing error may occur in April but may not necessarily be discovered until January of the following year when the patient files a lawsuit. The claim is then first made.

This differs from CGL policies, which are usually written on an occurrence basis. That is, the date a person is injured must occur during the policy period.

With claims made policies, the insurer may be exposed to a large number of claims arising out of the rendering of professional services several years before the inception date of the policy. Therefore, insurers have placed *retroactive dates* or *prior acts* limitations on the policies. A formal date (usually negotiable with the underwriter) prior to the inception date of the policy is set, whereby the policy will cover only claims made during the policy period that arise out of a medical incident that took place subsequent to this retroactive date.

Some insurers have taken the claims made concept one step further and have created a claims made and reported coverage. This means that the act must have taken place subsequent to the retroactive date and must be made against the hospital *and* reported to the insurer during the policy period.

A risk manager must carefully scrutinize the retroactive date at the time of purchase or renewal to be certain that no gaps for incident years will be created. He or she should also be aware of the relevant statute of limitations at the time the retroactive date is negotiated.

Finally, it is recommended that near the end of each claims made policy period, the risk manager should take an inventory of claims for that period to make sure of compliance with the claims made reporting requirement. Failure to do so may result in the denial of coverage for certain claims.

A broader discussion of claims made coverage and the differentiation between it and occurrence coverage may be found in Chapter 13.

POLICY FORMAT

Insurance policies contain certain provisions that are common to all of them:

1. declarations
2. insuring agreements/definitions
3. exclusions
4. conditions

Declarations

An insurance company issues its policy based on the declarations, or statements, of the insured. These statements, along with information gathered from other sources, allow the underwriter to issue the proper policy at a correct and competitive price.

One of the most important duties of a risk manager seeking coverage is to make certain that the correct information concerning the hospital appears on the policy's declarations page. The format of the declarations may vary from insurer to insurer, but it forms the bond of the contract. It clearly identifies the insurance company and the policy number it has assigned to the particular risk. Furthermore, it identifies the "named insured" and its status (i.e., corporation, partnership, nonprofit institution).

A risk manager must take a full inventory of all locations and facilities within a system at the time of application and be certain they are included in the "named insured" appearing in the declarations.

The policy limits, including any aggregates, and the policy period appear on this page. Finally, such items as the premium, types of coverage afforded, and retroactive date usually are stated on the declarations page.

Insuring Agreements and Definitions

The insuring agreement (coverage) distinguishes one coverage from another and defines the perils insured against. The insurer agrees that in consideration of the premium paid, it will provide protection in accordance with the provisions stated in the coverage part and any applicable endorsements.

The most critical portion for a risk manager to understand is the coverage section. It forms the basis for the insurer either to accept or deny coverage for a claim, based on the facts of the particular incident or occurrence. An incident or occurrence must always be reviewed in conjunction with the specific coverage provisions and the definitions of terms stated in the coverage.

The definitions section defines terms that are common to all or most coverage parts and policy provisions. They are usually highlighted as they appear in the text and are explicitly defined and explained in the definitions section.

Exclusions

No insurance policy covers all loss from the perils insured in the insuring agreements. All policies contain an exclusions section that states specifically what is *not* insured. Exclusions have three basic purposes:

1. They draw lines between the coverage of the policy and that afforded by other policies. For example, the CGL policy excludes injury to an insured arising out of employment, a peril that is covered by a workers' compensation policy.
2. They make exceptions that the insurer regards as uninsurable. One of the most common exclusions regarded as uninsurable is loss due to hostilities or warlike actions, to which are now being added nuclear energy hazards. Intentional acts are excluded because they are not accidental and often are against public policy.
3. They make exceptions to perils or risks that may be covered under the policy, but only after consideration by the underwriter and the payment of additional premium. These exclusions are removed by endorsement and allow the insured to extend its coverage at a higher expense.

The typical HPL policy contains a variety of exclusions. The most common three are

1. bodily injury to employees
2. liability arising out of the use of a motor vehicle, watercraft, or aircraft, excepting treatment given in an ambulance or other vehicle
3. personal liability of a staff member or employee

Conditions

A condition is a provision in the policy with which the insured must comply to enforce its rights under the policy. Conditions protect the interests of the carrier by requiring the insured to furnish timely information and to afford it the proper cooperation in the handling of claims and lawsuits.

A risk manager should pay special attention to meeting all conditions of the policy, especially where failure to do so will void the policy or where compliance must be on the initiative of the insured, such as the notification-of-claim condition. While detailed compliance is often not insisted upon, the risk manager and the insured ignore them at their own peril.

ENDORSEMENTS

Endorsements are riders that are added to the policy, usually to extend the coverage afforded. They supersede any provisions or terms with which they are in conflict in the basic policy. They must be clear and made a part of the policy if they are to be enforced. Endorsements serve many purposes, some of which are

- to change the limits of insurance
- to change or add locations
- to excuse the insured from a condition or exclusion stated in the policy
- to add additional insureds to the policy

REFERENCES

Anderson, Ronald A., and Walter A. Kumpf. *Business Law*. 9th ed. Cincinnati: South-Western Publishing Co., 1973.

F. C. & S. Bulletins. Cincinnati: The National Underwriter.

Gordis, Phillip. *Property and Casualty Insurance*. 23rd ed. Cincinnati: Rough Notes Co., 1974.

Miller, Jerome S., and C. Arthur Williams, Jr. *Insurance Principles and Practices: Property and Liability*. 6th ed. Englewood Cliffs, N.J.: Prentice-Hall Publishing Co., 1976.

Vaughan, Emmett J., and C.H. Elliott, *Fundamentals of Risk and Insurance*. Santa Barbara, Calif.: Wiley-Hamilton, 1972.

chapter 13

Understanding Claims Made Coverage: How It Differs from Occurrence Coverage

M. Michael Zuckerman

This chapter will explore the basic concepts of claims made coverage that distinguish it from occurrence liability insurance forms of coverage. As Chapter 12 mentioned, although occurrence coverage for hospital professional liability is difficult to purchase today, it continues to be available for comprehensive general liability. It is important to understand the differences between claims made and occurrence coverage, as often the risk manager will have to work with policies from prior years. This chapter is not intended to be a detailed examination of any particular primary or excess claims made liability insurance policy but rather an examination of the general principles that apply to purchasing either claims made or occurrence medical professional or general liability insurance coverage or to complying with the reporting requirements under each kind of policy. The key, however, to obtaining a thorough analysis of claims made versus occurrence coverage, as it applies to a particular insurance program, is to employ a competent insurance broker or consultant who can explain the strengths and weaknesses of such a program.

In the summer of 1984, the property casualty insurance industry was facing a financial crisis.[1] By the year's end this industry did incur record losses.[2] In fact, huge underwriting losses caused by underpriced policies, unwise investments of premiums, and larger than expected judgments generated by our legal system resulted in an after-tax loss of $2.09 billion in 1984.[3] Investment income could no longer make up for the huge underwriting losses being incurred by the industry.[4]

Increasing insurance premiums was not the only corrective action taken by the industry in 1985. The reintroduction of claims made insurance as the preferred form of coverage available for medical professional liability became commonplace. The London market and most notable domestic medical professional liability insurance carriers made the permanent shift to claims made coverage by abandoning their occurrence coverage forms altogether.

CLAIMS MADE AND OCCURRENCE COVERAGE DEFINED

To understand the development of claims made insurance, it is important to first define the concept of claims made and occurrence liability insurance forms. Occurrence coverage responds to events that occur during the policy year, regardless of when the claim is made. An occurrence policy written for a particular policy year will recognize any claim arising out of an event that occurred during that policy year, without regard for when the claim is ultimately brought. For example, an occurrence policy written for the 1989 policy year will cover claims brought up after this policy expires, as long as the event giving rise to the claim occurred during 1989. This creates what is known as a *tail exposure* for claims yet to be reported in the future for events that have already occurred.

Claims made insurance responds only to a claim made while the policy is in force. It does not recognize the date of the event per se. The policy's retroactive date, which will be discussed in greater detail later in this chapter, defines the point in time after which an event must occur in order for the claim arising therefrom to be covered by that policy. For example, a policy purchased for the year 1989 will recognize only claims brought in 1989. If an event occurred in 1988, but the claim is brought in 1990, the claim will not be covered by the claims made policy which was in force for 1988, as it would with an occurrence policy, even though the event occurred in 1988.

Claims made insurance is not a new concept. It has been around since the 1950s but was rarely used in the United States for medical professional liability insurance until the 1970s.[5] In fact, a major medical malpractice carrier in 1975 introduced claims made insurance to its physician policyholders. Directors' and officers' liability insurance is another professional liability coverage that has traditionally been written on a claims made form. At the beginning of the last hard insurance market, most professional liability insurance carriers that offered occurrence medical professional liability insurance policies converted to a claims made form, including the London insurance marketplace. There are some notable exceptions, such as a major domestic reinsurer (Employers Reinsurance Company), that still offer occurrence coverage for excess medical professional liability insurance; however, the price has risen dramatically. The London market in 1989 underwrites a significant amount of excess medical professional liability insurance for North American risks almost exclusively on a claims made form. (An excess liability insurance policy is one that pays for claims only after the applicable primary self-insurance or first-dollar insurance coverage has been exceeded, as recognized by the excess policy.)[6]

THE RETROACTIVE DATE

In order to fully understand the nature of claims made coverage, it is important to understand the concept of the retroactive date. The retroactive date is a point in time after which an incident must occur in order to be covered under a claims made policy. In other words, the event must occur after the retroactive date in order for any claim arising from that event to be covered by the current claims made policy. For example, assume the retroactive date stated on a current 1989 claims made policy is January 1, 1987. If an event occurs on February 1, 1987, but the claim arising from that event is not reported until February 1, 1989, it will be covered by the 1989 claims made policy limits.

To be more specific, the retroactive date defines the period of prior acts coverage. It defines which acts occurring prior to the effective date of the current claims made policy can give rise to claims that will be covered if reported under the current policy (sometimes referred to as *nose coverage*).

The retroactive date is usually the effective date of the first claims made policy placed with a new carrier. Therefore, there is usually no prior acts coverage under the first year of a claims made policy with a new carrier. As a result, the first year of the claims made program will be the least expensive because only claims arising out of events occurring after the inception date of the first-year claims made policy will be covered by the policy. This is because only approximately 26 percent of all claims that will arise out of events occurring in that first-year claims made policy period will actually be reported in the first year.[7] Therefore, a first-year claims made policy requires less premium, because the policy covers fewer claims than an occurrence policy will for the same period.

During the second year of the claims made policy, all claims reported in that policy year will be covered for events occurring over a two-year period of time (i.e., events occurring since the effective date of the first-year claims made policy). In turn, the third year of the claims made policy will cover a three-year occurrence period, which includes all claims arising out of events occurring since the original retroactive date, or the effective date of the first claims made policy. Therefore, as the program renews, it is of vital importance that the retroactive date is not advanced to each renewal date but remains the original effective date of the first claims made policy purchased from that carrier.

Purchasing claims made coverage for the first time creates certain problems for the insured. Since the effective date of the first year of a claims made policy is usually the retroactive date, there is no prior acts coverage under that policy. That being so, how will claims arising from these prior acts be covered? If the policy in force prior to the conversion to a first-year claims made policy form was occurrence coverage, then there is prior acts coverage for that policy year. In fact, if all the prior policies were occurrence policies, then claims arising from acts occurring during those policy years will be covered by the respective occurrence policies. Therefore, prior acts coverage is not an issue when the expiring program is an occurrence one.

On the other hand, if the insured is changing from one claims made insurance carrier to a new claims made insurance carrier, then the insured has two options: (1) purchase prior acts coverage from the new claims made carrier, if available (i.e., the new carrier honors the existing retroactive date of the expiring program) or (2) purchase tail coverage, which is an extended reporting period under the expiring policy, from the expiring claims made policy insurer, if it is available.

THE EXTENDED REPORTING PERIOD

An extended reporting period allows the insured to report claims against the expiring claims made insurance policy after it has expired. Specifically, the extended reporting period or tail provides coverage for events or acts that *occur* after a policy's retroactive date and prior to its expiration but that are *reported* as claims after the expiration of this policy, during the extended reporting period. The tail, therefore, could cover several years. There is usually an additional premium for this coverage, which usually is stated as a percentage of the expiring premium for the last claims made policy year.

The tail is needed if the insured or insurer cancels or "nonrenews" the claims made policy, coverage is modified to create a loss of coverage for some prior acts, the insured switches to occurrence coverage, the insured switches claims made insurers, or the retroactive date is advanced. In other words, when the current claims made coverage situation changes so that some or all prior acts that are presently covered will not be covered because of a change in terms at renewal, then a tail is necessary to provide coverage for those prior acts.

It is important to determine prior to binding coverage with any carrier under what conditions the insured will be able to purchase tail coverage if the policy is canceled or nonrenewed (i.e., what will trigger tail coverage). In other words, the insured must know when the right to exercise the extended reporting period or tail provision exists.

The most advantageous trigger for the insured is when the tail can be purchased when the policy is canceled or nonrenewed by either the insured or insurer or when there is any material change made in the current claims made insurance coverage by either the insured or insurer. The least advantageous trigger for the insured is when a tail can be purchased only if the insurer cancels or nonrenews the program. This leaves the insured in the position of not ever being able to leave a claims made carrier without having to assume the prior acts exposure or find a new insurer that will provide prior acts coverage.

An issue that arises under this worst case scenario is whether unreasonable renewal terms mean, in effect, nonrenewal on the part of the insurer. When the property and casualty insurance industry is in a soft market mode, an insured can anticipate fairly smooth renewals. What will happen when the market hardens again and claims made insurers demand unreasonable renewal terms? Will the insured be forced into self-insuring the prior acts exposure in order to find a new carrier that will offer more reasonable terms, or decide to self-insure the entire exposure, including prior acts?

The length of time for which claims may be brought under the tail is another point for negotiation. Pennsylvania, for example, requires that any primary claims made medical professional liability insurance policy sold must offer the option for the insured to purchase a tail regardless of who cancels or nonrenews the policy, for an unlimited period of time in the future. Oftentimes, excess liability insurance carriers will limit tail coverage to only one year. The insured must determine whether this is sufficient time to discover all claims or potential claims.

Excess claims liability insurance carriers are not as closely regulated as primary insurers. In Pennsylvania, for example, they are not required to offer an unlimited tail, as are primary insurers. An insurance buyer must, therefore, pay especially close attention to a claims made excess liability form that does not undergo the scrutiny of a state insurance department.

The Insurance Services Office (ISO) is an insurance industry-sponsored organization that develops insurance policies and rates for member companies. The ISO 1986 claims made commercial general liability policy form provides an example of various types of tail provisions. It offers an automatic 60-day tail period after the policy is canceled to report events that occur after the retroactive date but before the expiration of the last claims made policy in effect. If the claim is then brought within five years after reporting that event, it will be covered by this expiring policy.[8] This five-year extended reporting provision also applies to events reported during the policy year.[9] In addition, there is also an unlimited tail available for an additional premium under the new ISO claims made policy.[10]

The cost of a tail is of primary concern. Under the best conditions, the insured has prenegotiated the premium at the inception of the claims made policy. The more common situation is that the insurer uses a formula that calculates the tail premium as a percentage of the last expiring claims made annual premium. For example, a tail may cost up to 200 percent of the expiring annual premium. The worst case scenario is that the additional premium will be determined at the expiration of the claims made policy by the insurer. This leaves the insured subject to the conditions of the marketplace.

Some carriers, especially the excess liability insurance carriers, if they provide for a tail, will negotiate the premium for the tail only at the time it is purchased. Unfortunately, therefore, the insured has little opportunity to budget the funds necessary to cover the tail policy. It's always better to negotiate the cost of the tail at renewal so that the tail premium can be amortized over the life of the claims made insurance program. The cost of the tail will increase as the claims made program matures because the occurrence period covered also increases. Therefore, it is advisable to set aside the funds necessary to cover the cost of the tail prior to each renewal so that the insured has the financial ability to purchase the tail at the end of that particular claims made policy year. That fund should be augmented by the additional premium necessary to purchase the tail in each subsequent year as the claims made policy program matures.

Finally, the dollar limits of liability coverage available to the tail must be determined. The fundamental question is whether the original policy aggregate[11] limits of liability are reinstated for purposes of the tail or whether the impaired limits of the expiring claims made policy are converted to cover the tail period. Obviously, the best situation is a policy that reinstates the original policy aggregate limits of liability for the tail coverage period. If the limits of coverage available under the expiring claims made liability policy have been exhausted to pay claims already reported, then the insured must examine the amount of coverage available against the cost of the tail.

HOW IS A CLAIM DEFINED?

The insured must understand how the term "claim" is defined because it will determine how coverage is triggered under a claims made insurance policy. For example, does the definition of claims include incidents or events occurring during the claims made policy year, allowing them to be reported to the insurer as claims? Event or incident is defined here as a particular occurrence that has not yet given rise to an actual claim or demand for compensation but is the subject of coverage under the claims made liability insurance policy in question. Or does the policy define claims as only lawsuits or demands (written or oral) for compensation made against the insured during the policy year? Furthermore, if a claim is defined as a demand for compensation, must notification of this demand be sent to the insurer in writing during the claims made policy period? With occurrence form policies, the date of injury or event is the coverage trigger. Coverage under a claims made policy might also be secured by reporting the event even if the actual claim does not arise for several years.

Some claims made policies require that certain events or occurrences occurring during the policy period be reported to the underwriter. It is important to determine whether these events are reported simply for the underwriter's information or to guarantee or trigger coverage under the current claims made policy, in the event that a claim should arise in the future. Remember, claims made insurance is disappearing insurance. That is, once the policy expires, anything that has not been reported to that claims made policy year cannot be reported in the future unless an extended reporting period is purchased. Therefore, if permitted, reporting events under the current policy preserves coverage under limits of liability already purchased, in the event the claim is brought after the policy expires.

As a claims made program matures from a first- to a second-year claims made policy, claims not reported in the first year are then reported under the second year. The first year is forever closed for new claims. As previously stated, an exception is if the claims made policy allows the reporting of certain events as claims, as defined by the policy, during the first-year claims made policy year. If so, then coverage will be triggered under that first-year claims made policy year regardless of when the actual claim, if ever, is brought in the future. For example, if a medical professional claims made liability policy requires that the insured report the occurrence of all deaths (an event), the insured must determine whether this is for the underwriter's information only or for triggering coverage under the claims made policy regardless of when a claim is eventually brought. If the insured can report an event in order to trigger coverage and the claim arising from a reported death is not brought for several years following the date of event, then coverage will be found under the claims made policy year limits of liability in force when the event was originally reported. This event-reporting provision, in a sense, converts a claims made policy from pure claims made to a modified occurrence-type policy. It is therefore to the benefit of the insured to report events that trigger coverage, since you are securing coverage under policy limits for which a premium has been paid. If the policy expires with no claims or events reported to it in order to trigger coverage, then that coverage is forever gone, and those premium dollars have been lost.

A different issue is presented when the event-reporting requirement is for information only. The question is whether the underwriter by endorsement can exclude any future claims that arise from a particular event. Even if the reporting of an event does trigger coverage for any claim arising from that event, there still exists the possibility that an underwriter or renewal can use what is known as a laser endorsement[12] to exclude future claims arising from that event from being covered by future claims made policies.

Although the underwriter can use the laser endorsement to exclude all future claims arising from a specific reported event or occurrence, there may be a period of time allowed to report claims under that policy for which the event was reported. The other option available for the insured may be an unlimited extended reporting period endorsement, available to cover any claims arising from this excluded event. (ISO provides such an endorsement for its claims made commercial general liability form). The insurer has, in effect, limited all claims arising from this reported event to the policy limits of liability available under the policy for which the event was originally reported. On the other hand, if the insured ignores these information reporting requirements, then coverage could be jeopardized altogether.

Another issue related to informational event reporting that does not trigger coverage is whether the underwriter can advance the retroactive date in order to exclude claims being brought under future claims made policies that arise from these reported events, known activities, or products. Most insurers would agree that this type of action is, if not illegal, unethical. But it is a point that must be considered, especially if you are negotiating claims made general liability (as opposed to professional liability) coverage that does not follow the ISO 1986 claims made commercial general liability form and yet requires informational event reporting that does not trigger coverage. The ISO policy does require informational event reporting that does not immediately trigger coverage. However, even though coverage is not triggered, a retroactive date cannot be advanced under this ISO policy unless there is a change of insurers, the insured fails to provide material underwriting information, there is a material change in the exposure, or the insured requests it.[13] Therefore, under the ISO claims made commercial general liability form, the insured is protected against this type of action except under these few defined exceptions.

Once the insured determines the policy's event-reporting requirements, the sunset provision must be reviewed, if applicable. If the required event reporting does not immediately guarantee or secure coverage, the sunset provision requires that a claim arising from a reported event must be brought within a certain number of years of the date that the event was reported for there to be coverage under those policy limits. If the underwriter excludes claims arising from the reported event under future claims made policies, then there is still coverage under the policy for which the event was reported as long as the claim or claims arising from the event are then reported under the current policy within the sunset period. If the claim arises after the sunset period passes, then the insured has lost coverage. Some policy forms do not have sunset provisions and allow a claim to be filed regardless of when it is ultimately filed after the event has been reported for coverage-triggering purposes.

Many excess policies have sunset provisions, and these should be examined carefully. Sunset provisions often will vary according to whether they apply to general liability claims only or to hospitals' or physicians' professional liability claims as well.

Some occurrence policies also have event-reporting requirements and sunset provisions. Therefore, the insured should inquire about the existence of sunset provisions regardless of the form of coverage.

The final issue discussed here is whether the claim (actual demand for compensation) must be made orally or in writing against the insured only or whether it must be actually reported to the carrier during the claims made policy period. This presents a problem for the large firm where the designated individual (claims manager or risk manager) responsible for reporting claims to the carrier may not become aware that a claim has been filed against the firm within the claims made policy period. Therefore, this policy should be liberal enough (1) to recognize a claim as having been made during the policy period if it was filed against the firm during the policy period, and (2) to allow that it does not have to be reported to the carrier until received by a designated individual. The designated individual should be the risk manager or claims manager. Therefore, if a nondesignated individual is aware of a claim, the time period for reporting to the carrier to maintain coverage under the claims made policy year does not begin until the designated individual becomes aware of the claim.

The claims definition or coverage trigger concept can be best explained by example. The following series of events would occur following the purchase of a claims made medical professional liability insurance program with an effective date and retroactive date of July 1, 1984:

1. July 1, 1984: Retroactive date.
2. August 1, 1984: Service is provided by the health care provider to patient X.
3. July 1, 1985: Program is renewed as second-year claims made policy.
4. August 1, 1985: Injury is discovered and discussed with the health care provider. The event is reported to the insurer by the insured because it is an event that by definition must be reported to the carrier.
5. July 1, 1986: Program is renewed as third-year claims made policy.
6. August 1, 1986: Actual claim is filed by patient X and sent to the insurer.

If the policy provides for the triggering of coverage by reporting the event to the underwriter during the policy year, coverage will be provided by the claims made policy year 2, which began on July 1, 1985. If the claims made policy does provide for the reporting of events in order to trigger coverage, and there is a five-year sunset provision for the filing of a claim, then there still will be coverage under the second year's claims made policy because the claim was filed within the five-year period. If the claim had not been brought within that five-year sunset provision starting August 1, 1985, then there would be no coverage for that event. If the claims made policy did not permit the triggering of coverage by reporting an event not yet a claim, then coverage would, again, not be provided by the second-year claims made policy.

If coverage is triggered only by reporting the actual claim (demand for compensation) and not by reporting the event, then coverage will be provided by the claims made policy year 3, which began on July 1, 1986. By contrast, with the occurrence form of insurance, coverage will be provided by the policy year July 1, 1984/1985 because the event occurred during this period, on August 1, 1984.

It is helpful to compile checklists summarizing claims made policies' retroactive date(s), claim definitions, reporting requirements, tail coverage provisions, and costs for ready reference. Exhibit 13-1 shows a partial example of such a form.

THE PURPOSE OF CLAIMS MADE INSURANCE

Claims made insurance has made the purchasing of liability insurance more difficult, especially for the health care provider who has been forced

Exhibit 13-1 Partial Claims Made Policy Checklist

What Triggers Coverage?
Retroactive date, if any? _____
Claims made against:
 • insured only? _____
 • must notify insurer? _____
Claim in writing? _____
Event or incident reported to carrier is a
 claim? _____
Can the retroactive date be advanced?
 If so, how? _____
Extended Reporting Period
Can tail be purchased at insured's option?
If not, does a substantial change in renewal
 terms constitute nonrenewal? _____
Time limit for reporting claims for events
 already reported (sunset provision)? _____
Policy limits reinstated for tail coverage
 period? _____
Limited or unlimited period for reporting
 claims from known or unknown
 occurrences? _____
Is tail available for any changes in coverages,
 terms, or limits? _____
Cost:
Negotiated at policy inception _____
Percentage of expiring premium _____%
Other _____

into the claims made insurance market because of the nature of the medical professional liability exposure. It should at this point be more clear as to why claims made insurance has become the dominant form of coverage for professional liability. With the claims made form a liability insurer can more easily establish reserves because it knows that any claim or event reported during a particular policy year is the total number of claims that will be covered by that particular claims made policy year. The claims made policy form, unlike the occurrence form of coverage, is not exposed to a significant number of incurred but not reported claims at expiration for which reserves must be established. Therefore, the claims made concept brings more accuracy to the reserving process than is provided by occurrence coverage.

With claims made insurance, the insurer can limit its exposures to those claims already reported under the claims made policy, eliminating the tail exposure. This luxury is not available to the insurer under an occurrence policy. The occurrence policy remains exposed to all claims that arise at any time in the future from events occurring during the occurrence policy period.

The insurance industry has also instituted claims made insurance in reaction to the uncertainty created by the courts and our litigious society. The interpretation of what an occurrence is or what triggers coverage for occurrence insurance policies is often ruled by the desire to compensate an injured claimant, as opposed to what the insurance contract actually provides. An example of this is asbestos litigation where certain courts have held that all occurrence insurance contracts in force during the period of time over which an injured claimant is exposed to a specific hazard will be held to provide coverage if the exposure eventually causes injury.[14] This is known as the "exposure theory" for triggering liability insurance coverage and results in the stacking or combining of policy limits in force during the entire exposure period.[15]

In contrast to the exposure theory, the "manifestation theory" is preferred by insurers. The manifestation theory provides that the occurrence policy in force when the injury manifests itself must provide coverage. In certain cases, as cited above, the courts have ignored the manifestation theory in favor of the exposure theory, to engage more liability coverage for a particular event or situation. Again, claims made insurance is an attempt to limit this exposure since coverage is triggered only when the claims are filed, not when they occur.

This concept can be illustrated by re-examining our earlier example. If the service provided to patient X on August 1, 1984, was the prescription of a drug that was given continuously until a serious result manifested itself on August 1, 1985, there would be an issue as to which policy would provide coverage. Under the manifestation theory, assuming occurrence liability coverage, the policy providing coverage in 1985, the date the injury manifested itself, would be the policy called upon to provide coverage. Under the exposure theory, it would be those occurrence liability policies in force in 1984 and 1985 while the claimant was continuously exposed to the drug. This is an example of the stacking of policy limits from two occurrence policies in force during the exposure period, to provide twice the limits of coverage, which was not the intention of the insurer when the policies were issued.

Stacking is less possible with a claims made form. If the claims made policy provided for the triggering of coverage when an event is reported, then the policy in force on August 1, 1985, would provide coverage. If the claims made policy provided coverage only when an actual claim was made, then the policy in force in 1986 would provide coverage. The claims made insurer at renewal for 1987 could also exclude future claims arising from the administration of the drug in question, by use of a laser endorsement, to ensure that no future claims made policy limits of liability would be required to provide coverage. The insured must then explore the possibility of purchasing tail coverage for all future claims arising from the event if other patients were exposed to the drug, for example.

Insurers have also found themselves paying claims or portions of claims that at one time they were not responsible for. The concept of comparative negligence holds a defendant responsible for that amount of a claim that a jury can attribute as the insured's responsibility. As a result, the defense of contributory negligence no longer applies to free the defendant insured absolutely of financial responsibility, even if the claimant is partially responsible for her injuries. Joint and several liability is a legal concept that can hold a defendant liable for the full amount of a claim if the other defendants do not have the financial ability to pay their share of the claim. Finally, the concept of strict liability permits a claimant to pursue a products liability claim without having to prove the elements of ordinary negligence, making it easier to prove a claim. These concepts have exposed insurers who insure these defendants to a greater extent. Claims made insurance, especially for products liability and medical professional liability exposures, limits this uncertainty at least financially by restricting coverage to only those claims reported during the policy year. If the insurer then becomes uncomfortable with the risk, coverage can be canceled or excluded at renewal.

The results of this uncertain legal environment can be quantified. Medical professional liability claims costs have increased 150 percent from 1982 to 1986, with claims filed per 100 physicians increasing from 13.5 to 17.2 for the same time period.[16]

Medical professional liability, as previously mentioned, also creates a long tail exposure. With claims made insurance, an insurer can now charge a premium for the incurred but not reported claims exposure when it sells tail coverage or renews the policy. Some insurance carriers reserve the right to price the tail when it is exercised, on the theory that the price will be based on information known at the time the tail is exercised.

With all the advantages of a claims made liability policy format, it is unlikely that the insurance industry will revert back to occurrence coverage for the medical professional liability exposure.

There are some advantages for the insured, however, with claims made insurance. For example, the first claims made policy year is exposed to fewer claims and therefore should cost less than the comparable occurrence coverage. In fact, it should take several years for the claims made coverage to mature to the point that it costs the same as the occurrence policy form.[17]

Another advantage of claims made insurance is that the claims made limits of liability can be increased each year in relation to inflation or other related price indices, to ensure sufficient coverage for claims expected to be made in the upcoming policy year. With occurrence coverage the limits purchased for a policy year may be insufficient, due to inflation, to pay for claims brought several years following the expiration of the policy.

THE ADVANTAGE OF OCCURRENCE COVERAGE

Occurrence coverage is still the preferred insurance for health care providers. Occurrence coverage makes it easier to track claims. The insured knows that a claim is accounted for in an occurrence year by the date of event, not the date that the claim was reported or when the event was reported.

The need for tail coverage or prior acts coverage is also eliminated with occurrence coverage. The tail is covered on an unlimited basis without having to pay additional premium.

Event reporting under the claims made policy may also increase the insured's exposure to lawsuits if patients or plaintiffs or their legal counsel become aware that an insured has reported an event to its insurance carrier. The insured may be doing this simply because it is a condition to do so under its current claims made policy. The appearance, however, to a potential plaintiff is that the insured did something wrong and therefore has put its carrier on notice. In reality, the insured has merely identified an event that falls within the insurer's reporting requirements and is not necessarily the result of any negligence. With the traditional occurrence form of coverage, event reporting has not been an issue because the claim is attributed to whatever occurrence policy was in force at the time the event or occurrence occurred.

The insured, for example, must be aware of event reporting under the ISO 1986 occurrence commercial general liability policy form, which specifically requires that occurrences that may result in a claim must be reported to the underwriter. Nonetheless, the date of event still determines which occurrence policy provides coverage, as opposed to the date the event or claim was reported.

If an insured has purchased claims made general or professional liability coverage, it must note whether the policy defines the reporting of an event as a claim, that is, a coverage trigger. If this is the case, then, again, the insured is at risk that future claims arising from an occurrence or event could be excluded by advancing the retroactive date or by laser endorsement. Therefore, with claims made insurance the insured must understand the risk of losing coverage for events reported for informational purposes and what protections exist to avoid this risk.

AVOIDING GAPS IN COVERAGE BETWEEN PRIMARY AND EXCESS LIABILITY CLAIMS MADE PROGRAMS

It is incumbent upon any insured to understand the full impact of a claims made insurance form in order to avoid gaps in coverage created by layering one claims made policy on top of another to obtain the total necessary limits of coverage. To avoid these gaps, the retroactive date of the claims made program should be the same for all liability policies in force on the primary and excess liability insurance layers of the insured's program. That is, the retroactive date for the primary professional liability policy should be the same for the excess liability policies in force.

If the retroactive dates are not concurrent, then there is the creation of a gap in coverage. For example, if the claims made retroactive date for your primary layer is July 1, 1984, but your excess liability claims made retroactive date is July 1, 1986, how will the primary claims that go into the excess liability policy be covered for the period July 1, 1984, through July 1, 1986? Is there an excess occurrence form of coverage in place for those two years or, if not, was a tail purchased from the expiring claims made excess liability insurer for those years?

The definition of a claim for purposes of triggering coverage should be the same throughout the primary and excess liability program. Again, if coverage is triggered under the primary layer but not the excess layers, then there is the potential for a self-insured gap in coverage. Therefore, the insured must understand the definition of a claim under all the liability policies that make up the program.

With regard to tail coverage, does the excess coverage provide tail coverage to coincide with the primary coverage? Again, if the terms and conditions of the tail coverage are not concurrent, then there is a potential for gaps in coverage for claims falling within a tail period.

Finally, it is prudent that the effective date of each policy at each layer of your primary and excess liability insurance program be concurrent. This is true whether the coverage is occurrence or claims made. This will avoid a self-insured gap in coverage being created if the insured pays a claim on the primary level that occurred prior to the effective date of the excess policies and impairs the primary limit of liability. The excess carrier may not recognize this impairment of the primary limit because it occurred prior to its effective date. If this is the case, then a self-insured gap for the amount of the primary impairment has been created.

PROSPECTS FOR THE FUTURE

In 1988 there was some occurrence coverage available in the market-place, especially for excess medical professional liability insurance. One major domestic insurer that represents about half of the world's capacity for excess medical professional liability insurance coverage still provides occurrence coverage but usually over significant self-insured or insured primary insurance programs.

The London market, which represents the other major source of excess medical professional liability insurance coverage in the world, writes mostly on a claims made form. Also, a recent excess hospital professional liability captive insurer formed by several hospitals offshore opted for claims made rather than occurrence coverage.[18] Therefore, even hospitals are opting for claims made coverage for their own facilities.

On the primary level, claims made coverage is dominant for medical professional liability insurance even though occurrence coverage is still prevalent for other nonprofessional liability types of exposures. Most major domestic hospital professional liability insurance underwriters write only on a claims made form. This is a decision driven by the lack of available occurrence coverage from the reinsurance industry. This includes those carriers that write professional liability coverage for both hospitals and physicians.

Another example of the reduction in the availability of occurrence professional liability insurance coverage is on the primary level for physicians. In 1986 there were 33 physician-sponsored liability insurance companies, and 13 of them (40 percent) offered an occurrence product.[19] There is still some occurrence coverage available from physician-sponsored insurance carriers, but of approximately 41 physician-owned or sponsored insurance carriers in 1988, most wrote only claims made primary coverage for their physicians, due to reinsurance restrictions. Only about 8 companies (20 percent) now offer an occurrence product.[20]

Occurrence coverage has not completely disappeared in the hospital and physician professional liability marketplace. It has been significantly re-stricted, however. There is little prospect that either London or domestic carriers that write only claims made forms will shift back to occurrence coverage for this exposure, since such an event has yet to materialize in the current soft insurance market. Therefore, claims made insurance is a concept that will not go away for the medical professional liability exposure. It is a confusing concept, but one that must be mastered by risk managers.

NOTES

1. Insurance Information Institute, Insurance Facts: *1985–86 Property/Casualty Fact Book* (New York: Insurance Information Institute, 1985), p. 6.

2. Ibid.

3. Ibid.

4. Ibid.

5. Myron F. Steves, "Medical Professional Liability," in *Professional Liability: Impact in the Eighties*. The Society of Chartered Property and Casualty Underwriters, ed. (Malvern, Pa.: The Society of Chartered Property and Casualty Underwriters, 1983), p. 97.

6. Harvey W. Rubin, *Dictionary of Insurance Terms* (New York: Barrons Publishing Co., 1987), p. 96.

7. Myron F. Steves, "Medical Professional Liability," p. 98.

8. See International Risk Management, "Coverage Triggers," in *Commercial Liability Policies*, vol. 2 (Dallas: International Risk Management Institute, 1988), pp. C.11–12.

9. Ibid., pp. C.9–C.11.

10. Ibid., pp. C.13–C.14.

11. Many liability policies state dollar limits available to pay claims as per occurrence or annual aggregates. If the policy has an aggregate limit, then there is a cap on the total amount a policy will pay for claims in any one year, regardless of the number of occurrences.

12. See International Risk Management, "Coverage Triggers," pp. C.17–26.

13. See International Risk Management, "Coverage Triggers," pp. C.6, 7.

14. International Risk Management, "Products Liability in Longterm Exposure Cases," *The Risk Report* 6, no. 10 (June 1984): 6.

15. International Risk Management Institute, "Claims-made Insurance," *The Risk Report* 8, no. 8 (Apr. 1986): 2.

16. Insurance Information Institute, *Insurance Facts: 1988–89 Property/Casualty Fact Book* (New York: Insurance Information Institute, 1988), p. 59.

17. Myron F. Steves, "Medical Professional Liability," p. 98.

18. Janet Aschkenasy, "Hospitals Turn to Captive for Excess Coverage," *National Underwriter* (Property and Casualty/Employee Benefits Edition), Feb. 9, 1987, p. 6.

19. Information provided November, 1988, courtesy of the PMSLIC Insurance Company. PMSLIC is a physician-sponsored company owned by the Pennsylvania Medical Society.

20. Ibid.

REFERENCES

Aschkenasy, Janet. "Hospitals Turn to Captive for Excess Coverage." *National Underwriter* (Property and Casualty/Employee Benefits Edition), Feb. 9, 1987, p. 6.

Breslin, Paul H. "Checklist for Using the Claims Made CGL Form." *Risk Management* 33, no. 10 (Aug. 1986): 25–26.

Clark, Brant R. "The Broad Implications of Claims-made Insurance." *Risk Management Reports* 13, no. 4 (July/Aug. 1986): 9–33.

Herrick, R.C. "Effects of the New CGL: Do Your Contracts Still Mean What They Say?" *Risk Management* 33, no. 3 (Mar. 1986): 25–34.

Insurance Information Institute. *Insurance Facts: 1985–86 Property/Casualty Fact Book*. New York: Insurance Information Institute, 1985.

———. *Insurance Facts: 1988–89 Property/Casualty Fact Book*. New York: Insurance Information Institute, 1988.

International Risk Management. "Coverage Triggers." In *Commercial Liability Policies. Vol. 2*. Dallas: International Risk Management Institute, 1988.

———. "Products Liability Coverage in Long Term Exposure Cases." *The Risk Report* 6, no. 10 (June 1984): 1–7.

International Risk Management Institute. "Claims-Made Insurance." *The Risk Report* 8, no. 8 (Apr. 1986): 1–8.

———. "Insurance Market Report." *The Risk Report* 10, no. 1 (Sept. 1987): 1–8.

Lavertue, Anna. "Occurrence or Claims-Made—What's the Difference." *The PMSLIC Pulse* 6, no. 4 (Winter 1988): 2.

Lincoln, Victor D. "Liability Exposure and the Claims-Made Concept." *CPCU Journal* 39, no. 4 (Dec. 1986): 224–33.

Robertson, James A. "Making the New Umbrellas Fit the New CGL." *Risk Management* 33, no. 8 (Oct. 1986): 18–30.

Rubin, Harvey W. *Dictionary of Insurance Terms*. New York: Barrons Publishing Co., 1987.

Shand, Morahan & Company, Inc. "The Effect of the New ISO Claims Made Form on Professional Liability Insurers." Evanston, Ill.: Shand, Morahan & Company, Inc., Apr. 1986, pp. 1–4.

Steves, Myron F. "Medical Professional Liability." *Professional Liability: Impact in the Eighties*. Malvern, Pa.: The Society of Chartered Property and Casualty Underwriters, 1983, pp. 91–103.

PART V

Management of Actual and Potential Claims

Maintaining the financial integrity of the institution is one of the primary responsibilities of the risk management department. Accomplishing this goal is closely tied with the risk manager's ability to successfully monitor and manage claims. A great deal of expertise must be developed before a risk manager will be successfully able to identify risk, intervene early, monitor potential incidents and manage claims and lawsuits.

The purpose of Part V is to assist the risk manager with gaining expertise in all of the aspects of risk identification and loss control. Reviewed in Part V is the development of a system to (1) identify risk and effectively report it, (2) follow up and monitor the reports filed, (3) set up claim files, and (4) handle files through the initial investigation, discovery, and litigation phases.

chapter 14

The Importance of Early Identification in the Claims Management Process

A. Michele Kuhn

Hospital risk management presents a difficult and challenging task to the experienced risk manager who is new to the hospital environment, as well as to the hospital employee newly appointed to the risk management position. Unlike the industrial risk manager, whose primary interest is the financial status of the organization, the hospital risk manager is also concerned with the quality of patient care. Hospital risks can be successfully managed and the quality of care improved through the application of sound risk and claims management principles. The first step in this process and clearly the most important is risk identification. Risk identification is the collection of information that alerts the risk manager to a situation that presents a potential or actual loss to the hospital. In order to be successful in this process of identification, the risk manager has to overcome the resistance of the medical staff and hospital personnel to becoming involved. There is a natural tendency for physicians and health care professionals to be very defensive about the care they render, and recognizing that fact is critical to the risk manager's success in involving these key persons in the process.

Early identification of risks is important for several reasons:

1. Potential problems with procedures can be identified, and corrections can be made before another incident occurs.
2. Possible equipment defects can be identified, and the equipment can be repaired or put out of circulation.
3. Investigation can be implemented while the occurrence is fresh in the mind of the person involved.

4. Possible action can be taken in the form of a reimbursement to the patient or a hospital charge write-off, before the patient becomes angry and takes further legal action.

The methods of identifying risks that will be discussed in this chapter are

1. maintaining open lines of communication
2. trending risks by analyzing incident reports and the hospital's loss experience
3. integrating operations with quality assurance
4. monitoring patient correspondence and complaints
5. investigating complaints lodged with the hospital's credit department
6. keeping tabs on attorney requests for records
7. analyzing regulatory agency surveys
8. making recommendations on contracts negotiated with outside firms
9. attending committee meetings
10. attending hospital rounds

The risk management department can utilize all of these methods but will not necessarily be limited to them.

MAINTAINING OPEN LINES OF COMMUNICATION

The first step, basic to this process of identification and one that must take place in order to utilize any of the other steps, is ensuring open lines of communication. Establishing and maintaining open lines of communication are the most effective methods of identifying risks. In order to establish a line of communication, employees and medical staff must be made aware of the concept of risk management and its purpose of protecting both staff and patients. This is best accomplished through lectures or informal talks to at least the following five orientation groups (for more detailed discussion of the value and process of staff education, see Chapter 7):

1. new employees
2. nurses
3. management
4. medical staff
5. medical residents (in a teaching hospital)

Presentations to these regularly scheduled groups are essential. However, even more important is the ongoing educational process. The risk manager must set as one of the goals of the risk management department frequent presentations to different patient units' and hospital departments' staff and medical staff. Because hospitals are operational 24 hours a day, it will also be necessary to schedule presentations on the off-hour shifts, to accommodate professional staff who work evenings and nights.

The content and method of presentation will influence how the information is received by staff. Following a presentation, an employee should

1. understand the concept of risk management
2. know the purpose of an incident report or an initial investigation report
3. understand the importance of reporting
4. know the methods of reporting and how to properly complete a report
5. feel comfortable that reporting an incident will not result in punitive action
6. understand that negative situations result in additional cost to the hospital
7. recognize that one of the goals of risk management is to enhance the quality of care provided
8. expect feedback and action regarding a reported occurrence

Feedback is critical to keeping lines of communication open. Employees who perceive that no action has taken place following an observation made by them will cease to be a source of information.

The risk manager must practice effective listening. This takes time, but employees who are confident that the risk manager will listen to their observations and offer assistance are more likely to communicate on a regular basis and to provide the risk manager with sensitive information.

When timely feedback and effective listening are practiced, the risk manager will gain staff compliance and greatly increase the likelihood of early reporting. You will see as you go on that all of the following methods of identification relate back to this first step.

TRENDING RISKS

Incident and Initial Investigation Reports

Probably the most widely known and recognized method of identification is the incident report or the initial investigation report. "Initial investigation report" (IIR) is considered a more appropriate term because everything that is reported is not necessarily an incident; only after an investigation will the risk manager recognize the implications of the report. The IIR is a valuable tool to the risk manager, and it has no real counterpart in other industrial settings. Hospital staff are required to generate a report upon the occurrence of any happening that is not consistent with the routine operation of the hospital or the routine care of the patient. Incident reports often provide the risk manager with information regarding "low exposure, low liability" occurrences, but the more sensitive the monitoring tool and the more familiar staff are with the process and with risk management staff, the greater the likelihood that significant problems and behaviors will be reported. Basic subject areas to include on the initial investigation report are

1. falls
2. medication
3. surgical procedures
4. radiology procedures
5. blood administration
6. patient care/general
7. equipment
8. physical plant
9. small claims
10. miscellaneous

There are, of course, subheadings under each of these, and other areas may be included, depending on the hospital and its specialty. An example of an initial investigation report and the information it should contain are shown in Exhibit 14-1.

The risk manager needs to encourage health care professionals and physicians to verbally report what they do not have time to write a report about or feel hesitant to report. Many times a physician does not have the time to write a report but does want to alert the risk manager to a potential problem or perceived problem with the care of one of his or her patients. Effective listening and feedback to the physician can result in the establishment of an important source of information. The physician will learn to rely on the risk manager for correction or resolution of a problem and at the same time realize the importance of early investigation.

The same is true of any health care professional. Nurses may not always be sure if a report is necessary when a patient's family is issuing complaints but will welcome the opportunity to communicate this to the risk manager.

When a report is delivered verbally, the risk manager should complete the written form for inclusion in the database. It is a good idea to develop a list of questions to ask such callers. An example of this type of list is shown in Exhibit 14-2. Gathering this information on the initial call will

Exhibit 14-1 Initial Investigation Report

NAME _____ UNIT _____
        LAST   FIRST   MIDDLE
                  (PLEASE PRINT)
MEDICAL RECORD NUMBER _____   SEX ___ M ___ F   AGE _____
CURRENT MEDICAL PROBLEM _____   _____   DATE OF INCIDENT ___/___/___
SERVICE/ATTENDING   TIME OF INCIDENT
PHYSICIAN _____   _____ A.M. _____ P.M.

IDENTIFICATION	**EXACT LOCATION OF OCCURRENCE (check 1)**	
☐ a Inpatient	☐ a Ambulating	☐ g Operating Room No. ___
☐ b Outpatient	☐ b G.I. Lab	☐ h Patient Room No. _____
☐ c Visitor	☐ c Occup. Therapy	☐ i Pt. Bathroom No. _____
☐ d Student	☐ d Physical Therapy	☐ j Radiology Room No. ___
☐ e Volunteer	☐ e Lounge No. _____	☐ k Other _____
☐ f Other _____	☐ f Lobby/Floor No. _____	

PATIENT'S CONDITION BEFORE INCIDENT	**IF INCIDENT OCCURRED IN PATIENT'S ROOM, CHECK DEPARTMENT INVOLVED**	
☐ a Normal	☐ a Admissions	☐ h Nursing
☐ b Impaired	☐ b CLIS	☐ i Pharmacy
☐ c Disoriented	☐ c Dietary	☐ j Physical Therapy
☐ d Sedated	☐ d EEG	☐ k Plant Services
☐ e Unknown	☐ e Housekeeping	☐ l Radiology
☐ f Pt. Was Restrained	☐ f House Staff	☐ m Respiratory Therapy
	☐ g Medical Staff	☐ n Social Services
		☐ o Other _____

_____

_____

_____

NAME OF PHYSICIAN NOTIFIED _____ N/A _____
                                                         ___/___/___
SIGNATURE OF PERSON COMPLETING   TITLE   DATE OF REPORT

PATIENT AWARE
OF OCCURRENCE   ☐ Yes   ☐ No
PATIENT/FAMILY AWARE OF
OCCURRENCE   ☐ Yes   ☐ No
PATIENT/FAMILY
THREATEN SUIT   ☐ Yes   ☐ No
OTHER, PLEASE SPECIFY _____

_____

PATIENT'S CONDITION FOLLOWING OCCURRENCE   PHYSICIAN COMMENTS/TX

☐ a Unchanged	☐ f Infection
☐ b Burn	☐ g Laceration/Cut	_____
☐ c Concussion	☐ h Strain
☐ d Death	☐ i Other	_____
☐ e Fracture	

                                                          ___/___/___
PHYSICIAN SIGNATURE   DATE

   NOTE: This form is not a part of the patient's medical record.
NOTIFY the Risk Manager if the incident is serious.

Source: Courtesy of Presbyterian-University Hospital of Pittsburgh, Pittsburgh, Pennsylvania.

Exhibit 14-2 Information Sheet

```
 1. Patient's Name _____
 2. Record Number _____
 3. Unit/Ward Number _____
 4. Age _____
 5. Occupation _____
 6. Marital Status _____
 7. Dependents _____
 8. Insurance Company _____
 9. Admission Diagnosis _____
10. Date of Occurrence _____
11. Nurses _____
    _____
12. Attending Physician _____
13. Residents _____
14. Anesthesiologist _____
15. Surgical Procedures _____
16. Complications of Admission _____
    _____
    _____
17. Incident Report Filed: Yes _____ No _____
18. Verbal Report _____
19. Establish File _____
20. Board Report _____ Month _____
```

eliminate the need to call the physician or nurse back and, more important, will give the risk manager a head start on the investigation.

The incident report or the IIR on an individual basis may not be of significant value to the institution unless it reports an occurrence involving a serious injury. However, compiling these reports and trending them will identify potential risks in the hospital.

Employees often ask why they are required to complete a report for what they consider a minor occurrence. An example might be the administration of medicine X instead of medicine Y. The risk manager must emphasize to employees that although a minor incident may occur "only once" in their department/unit/ward, it may also occur "only once" in every other department/unit/ward and that the total number of times it occurs is the significant factor. The risk manager identifies this trend when reviewing each report and through the monthly statistics. The reason for this specific incident might be that the packaging for the medication is similar and therefore confusing to those who administer it. This incident could then be followed up by the hospital pharmacy and corrective action could be taken.

The trending may reveal that patient falls occur more on the evening shift or that medication errors occur most frequently at the end of a shift. When a trend is identified, the risk manager reports this to the appropriate personnel for corrective action.

A good example of the value of trending is in the following story: A special bed was being used to reduce infection in patients with wounds. However, within a short time period there were six incidents reported (from different patient units) relating problems with patients falling between the mattress and the side of the bed, along with other minor issues. These incidents from six different areas were brought to the attention of the appropriate person in the nursing department by the hospital's risk analyst. The result of the investigation was discontinuation of the use of the special bed. The manufacturer, however, responded to the problems identified and to the potential for a more serious occurrence and immediately instituted modifications to the equipment. In addition, the manufacturer agreed to take into consideration other recommendations of the nursing staff and the risk manager and undertook additional modifications. This is an example of identification, trending, follow-up, corrections, and then, of course, the monitoring stage.

Keep in mind the importance of early investigation of an incident (discussed in greater detail in Chapter 16). Usually a period of time passes (depending on your state's statute of limitations) between the incident's occurrence and the filing of a malpractice suit. Personnel may not recall the incident after a protracted length of time, and thus there is great value to be gained from early identification and investigation. It is important to interview staff when the incident is fresh in their minds.

When an incident is identified by one department of the hospital, it needs to be addressed and answered by the appropriate person in the department involved in the incident. An easy way to accomplish this is by sending a follow-up investigation form (Exhibit 14-3) to the department for its response. The department of origination should be sent a copy of the response. The most important part of this process is the feedback it provides, which reinforces the fact that action has been taken on a reported problem and that employee input is valued.

Hospital Loss Experience Data

The risk manager should enter claims and legal suits into the trending database. The hospital's loss experience is a significant area of risk identification to the risk manager. Problems encountered during the investigation of a claim should receive the same attention as any incident report.

Exhibit 14-3 Follow-Up Memorandum Regarding an Incident Report

---

TO:

FROM: Risk Analyst

DATE:

SUBJECT: ATTACHED INCIDENT REPORT
            INCIDENT REPORT #

The attached incident report is to be investigated by you and/or the responsible person in your department.

Please report your findings and make recommendations regarding corrective or preventive measures that will be taken.

Return the copy of the incident report, along with your comments, to the Risk Management Office within seven days.

Thank you for your cooperation.

KC/caf
Enclosure

Follow-up investigation, correction, and monitoring must occur, to reduce the risk of the same claim occurring again. More important, by reviewing and analyzing claims, the risk manager can eliminate risk to the patient and improve the quality of care to all patients. (This process is discussed in greater detail in Chapter 18.)

A lawsuit provides the risk manager the opportunity to identify policy and procedure deficiencies, documentation problems, communication gaps between medical staff and hospital personnel, and any number of other issues. The risk manager has to be involved in all processes related to the filing of a lawsuit. This involvement can consist of

1. investigating the incident immediately
2. responding to interrogatories
3. attending depositions of medical staff and hospital personnel
4. establishing reserves
5. attending the trial

Following the conclusion of a lawsuit, whether by settlement or verdict, the risk manager and the defense counsel handling the case need to summarize all relevant aspects of the suit. This summary should include the problems encountered and the reasons why the suit had to be settled. The issues identified need to be brought to the attention of the physician and hospital staff involved. The risk manager should follow up at a later date to determine if corrective action has taken place.

INTEGRATING OPERATIONS WITH QUALITY ASSURANCE

The risk manager and the quality assurance coordinator must share their data to have an effective risk management and quality assurance program. The quality assurance coordinator may identify problems that have not been reported to the risk manager, in the course of reviewing patient charts. The risk manager in turn shares the data gathered on trends in patient care with the quality assurance coordinator.

Follow-up and corrective actions taken as a result of quality assurance involvement should also be included with the risk management data.

MONITORING PATIENT CORRESPONDENCE AND COMPLAINTS

Typically, letters from patients or the hospital's patient representatives, containing either positive or negative comments, are sent to either the chief executive or the administrator of the hospital, the patient relations representative, the marketing division (through a survey), a specific department, or a nursing unit. The risk manager should establish a system whereby copies of all correspondence are sent to the risk management office. Staff should understand that letters from patients or patients' representatives may be answered by the appropriate personnel, but that if they involve any perceived or real problem with patient care, specifically a problem that alleges injury to the patient, the response to the patient must be approved by the risk manager. The risk manager should control any monetary reimbursement to or settlement with the complainant. Depending upon the insurance program your hospital is associated with, decisions regarding settlement of a claim will probably need to be discussed and coordinated with a representative of the insurance company. A settlement with the patient or a bill "write-off" could affect any subsequent claim; the implications of such action should be discussed with defense counsel.

Correspondence from a patient or a patient's representative most likely will not be the risk manager's first notification of a potential claim. The information known to the risk manager is important to the person responding to the complaint. Again, the early identification of a problem will assist the risk manager in the decision-making process.

Risk managers should work closely with the patient representatives of their hospitals. Although "patient reps" are primarily patient advocates, they are aware of the importance of potential liability issues. A good working relationship with the patient representatives serves two purposes for the hospital. First, the patient's complaints are addressed in an expedient manner, with possible reimbursement or settlement when applicable. This results in "happy" patients and satisfied customers. Second, potential liability issues are identified early, and resolution is possible before a problem escalates to a legal suit.

Another valuable source of information regarding patients' perceptions and concerns is the social worker. The risk manager must establish a working relationship with the social workers in the hospital so that they understand that he or she is a resource for any problems they encounter. They can also assist in identifying possible risks in the hospital or patient claims.

INVESTIGATING CREDIT DEPARTMENT ACTIVITIES

One of the top motivators of lawsuits is money. This is not only the money patients think they might be awarded if they are successful with their litigations, but also the money they owe to the hospital that they wish to avoid paying.

Patients may have a routine admission and be satisfied customers until they receive a bill from the hospital for services not covered by their insurance policies. If they do not have insurance coverage, the magnitude of the bill may cause them to seek remuneration for "less than perfect" service.

Patients may call the credit department and tell the account representative why they do not believe they should have to pay the amount due. This story could involve the patients' perceptions of the level of care administered or be a complaint about the food or housekeeping services. Whatever the reason, it is important that the employee in the credit office be aware of the risk manager's role and alert him or her to any allegation of negligence. The risk manager has to follow up by reviewing these patients' charts, talking with nursing staff involved in their care, and talking with the patients' physicians.

Staff involved will provide valuable information to help in making a decision. During the investigation of such a case, arrangements should be made with the credit office to "hold" the patient's bill until you advise them otherwise. Do not ignore a patient's complaint because on the surface it seems insignificant; you may find that a patient complaining about a communication gap with the physician has in fact suffered a complication. The results of your follow-up investigation will determine what you recommend to the credit office. Again, any decision to write off or forgive a bill or portion of a bill should be made in conjunction with the hospital's insurer and legal counsel. The hospital's legal counsel should advise you regarding a release statement that the patient should be asked to sign. A possible alternative to a release is to have a statement regarding "full and final settlement" typed on the check issued to the claimant. If your decision involves a question about the physician's care of the patient, you should consult the physician and respect his or her judgment as to whether a charge should be forgiven.

If the decision is made to discontinue billings, this does not mean that the risk manager will never see that patient's name again. A file should be established and monitored for further legal action. Of course, the ideal is for this good faith gesture to satisfy the client, so that he or she is never heard from again. Good documentation should be kept in the file regarding the write-off process, in the event that a suit is initiated.

MONITORING ATTORNEY REQUESTS FOR RECORDS

Attorneys request patient medical records for review when they are deciding whether to accept a case for litigation. The attorney sends the request not only to the medical records department but also to all of the departments that have participated in the patient's care. Physicians may also receive an attorney request for records.

A system needs to be established so that the risk manager is notified of these requests. The most efficient system is to have copies of all letters of request sent to the risk manager. Some letters specifically note the caption of the suit or give the reason for the request, and these may be disregarded (if they relate to third-party insurance interests and not to possible negligence). Any others should be submitted to the appropriate department with a request to review the record. A suggested form to use when reviewing the record is shown in Exhibit 14-4. The purpose of the review is not to do an in-depth investigation and analysis but rather to look briefly at the chart to determine if there is an obvious reason for the attorney request, such as an accident, a workers' compensation claim, a social security claim, or a claim against another hospital.

Exhibit 14-4 Medical Record Review Form

Memorandum

TO:

FROM: Risk Manager

SUBJECT: Attorney Request for Records List

DATE:

Please pull the following charts on ————————————————— for my review.
Thank you.

PATIENT NAME   RECORD NUMBER   ATTORNEY

NATURE OF CHART

NATURE OF CHART

NATURE OF CHART

NATURE OF CHART

NATURE OF CHART

NATURE OF CHART

NATURE OF CHART

NATURE OF CHART

Medical records that do not reveal an obvious reason for a request need to be searched further for the following:

1. an unexpected complication incurred by the patient
2. an unexpected readmission to the hospital
3. an infection acquired in the hospital (nosocomial infection)
4. an extended admission
5. an emergency department visit with no obvious explanation and the patient's being discharged

When it has been determined that there is a possible claim, a file should be established, and legal action should be monitored.

If the risk manager's other methods of identification are successful, a claim file will already be established when the attorney request for records is received. This request should be added to the file, and the hospital's attorney should be alerted so he or she can begin or continue an investigation.

ANALYZING REGULATORY AGENCY SURVEYS

Hospitals undergo surveys and audits by a number of regulatory agencies and sometimes by their insurance companies. These surveys should be considered by the risk manager as another method to identify potential areas of risk. In the course of an audit, the representatives of the surveying agency may identify areas of risk that have not been reported by the hospital staff and have gone unnoticed by the risk manager. The agency's recommendations should be reviewed, investigated, referred to the appropriate department for follow-up, and monitored for any trends.

This method of identification is different from the previously discussed methods in that it identifies areas of risk prior to a claim. This gives the risk manager the opportunity to work with other hospital staff to correct a problem before it leads to an incident. Employees should be encouraged to complete "hazard" reports to identify potential problems. The IIR form can be used for this purpose. Department-specific clinical indicators (discussed in Chapters 4 and 5) also serve to identify high-risk areas or behaviors prior to injuries occurring.

In this category, peer review organizations (PRO) can also be considered a means of identification of problems with care rendered. If a PRO refuses payment because of substandard care, the risk manager should be made aware of this refusal and then initiate a review of the record. The risk manager and utilization review nurses of the hospital should work together in determining potential claims.

The Joint Commission on Accreditation of Healthcare Organizations (Joint Commission) establishes guidelines for hospitals, which are published in its *Accreditation Manual for Hospitals*. Hospitals, of course, strive to meet these standards and undergo Joint Commission surveys to determine their compliance with them. The risk manager should use the report generated by the Joint Commission as a risk identification tool. In addition, the accreditation manual establishes the minimum standards a hospital must meet; the risk manager should know the manual and ensure that departments are in compliance with it.

PARTICIPATING IN OUTSIDE CONTRACT NEGOTIATIONS

This is another method of identification allowing the risk manager to identify a potential problem and correct it before it escalates to a claim. Whether the hospital has in-house counsel or uses an outside firm, the risk manager should be involved in the contract review process. Contracts for outside services include, or should include, a clause relating to the insurance provisions. The limits of insurance should be decided on by each risk manager, according to state regulations and individual institutions' decisions. The risk manager will review and determine the following:

1. What are the limits required of the contracted service?
2. Is the hospital named as an additional insured?
3. Does the service contracted for involve additional or unusual risk to the hospital?
4. Does the hospital have the ability and right to monitor and evaluate the quality of the contract service provided?

The risk manager should recommend to administration the appropriate action for monitoring and maintaining the quality of the contracted service.

ATTENDING COMMITTEE MEETINGS

The risk manager or a member of the risk management staff should participate in *at least* the following committees:

1. infection control
2. patient care
3. hospital safety
4. patient safety

In addition, the minutes from other committees should be made available to the risk manager for review. If the risk management staff is too small to act as members of many committees, then the risk manager should propose attending the committee meetings on a quarterly basis to present statistics relevant to that committee. This quarterly presentation will remind committee members of the importance of the risk management function. Other committees that it would be helpful to be a member of are

- critical care
- pharmacy and therapeutics
- emergency department
- medical records
- operating room

ATTENDING HOSPITAL ROUNDS

Because a risk manager's schedule is always full, it helps to designate a time every week when hospital rounds will be made. Rounds should include all areas of the hospital. They serve as a method for identifying potential hazards and risks, but, more important, they give the risk manager the opportunity to talk with nursing staff, department heads, and medical staff on an informal basis. Seeing the risk manager on the patient unit may jog a physician's memory about an occurrence. It is somehow much easier to talk to someone in person than to write a note or make that phone call. Such "visiting" opens lines of communication and increases staff's awareness of the risk management function.

In addition to hospital rounds, the risk manager or his or her staff should be available as a resource to hospital employees on a 24-hour basis. If the risk management staff is small, an answering machine or service should be used to allow callers to leave messages. The risk manager should carry a pager during the working hours, and the hospital operator should have a home phone number for the risk manager.

The risk manager's willingness to act as a resource will increase the willingness of medical and hospital staff to report occurrences.

RISK MANAGEMENT ACTION REPORT

It is a good idea to establish a mechanism for reporting and recording the action taken to correct identified risks. Exhibit 14-5 gives an example

Exhibit 14-5 Risk Management Action Report

<table>
<tr><td>

Risk Management/Problem Identification & Assessment

1. Description of Problem or Concern:

2. How Identified:

3. Assessment:

4. Action Taken:

Problem reviewed by: _____ Date: _____

</td></tr>
</table>

of a report suitable for this. This report accomplishes two purposes: (1) It provides a mechanism to track and trend any future incidents of the same nature, and (2) it provides the risk manager with documentation of corrective actions.

This report is filled out for any incident trend identified and is updated as the incident recurs. The follow-up investigation and the action taken are noted, and then any subsequent incidents of the same nature are noted on the report. If the incident continues to occur, the risk manager needs to develop a more aggressive approach to handling the situation. To establish the mechanism to handle recurring problems it is important that the risk manager

1. meet with the appropriate personnel and attempt to learn why the incident has recurred and the personnel's suggestions for prevention
2. review the corrective action initially taken, with an emphasis on analysis of why this action failed
3. recommend additional changes and a plan for their implementation

This report also serves as documentation for the risk management annual report detailing results of action taken during the year.

CONCLUSION

Unidentified risks cannot be analyzed or resolved; therefore, the risk is retained and unfunded. This unidentified risk creates a potentially dangerous situation that could affect the financial stability of the hospital.

The risk management function is a team effort that must focus on the importance of the early identification of all actual and potential risks. The risk manager must obtain the cooperation of all hospital personnel, and this cooperation can often best be gained by emphasizing the link between early identification of injury and development of a quality program focusing on providing a safe, healthy environment. Every person in the hospital has a role to play in risk management activities. The identification process can be a very easy one for the risk manager if an open line of communication is established and feedback to the personnel involved is practiced.

chapter *15*

Setting Up a Claim File and Protecting the Information

M. Ross Oglesbee

Hospital risk management programs, to be effective, must receive accurate, candid information from hospital employees about adverse patient care occurrences. In order for this to occur, a flexible and simple incident reporting system must be in place to promote prompt reporting. Letters addressed to the risk manager or hospital attorney and verbal reports received over the telephone or in person by risk management staff should be accepted methods of reporting incidents. If possible, the hospital should install 24-hour recording equipment so that reports by telephone may be called in and recorded any time, day or night, weekend or holiday. In addition, the hospital should design an incident reporting form that promotes the documentation of factual, necessary information. Of critical importance is a system in which all reports, in whatever form, receive careful evaluation and appropriate investigation and management while being treated in a confidential manner. This chapter will discuss the principles of confidentiality pertaining to hospital incident reports, the initial investigation process as it relates to obtaining information to establish a claim file, and the initial steps related to claims management.

POLICY AND PROCEDURE ON REPORTING INCIDENTS

Hospitals should develop policies and procedures consistent with the primary purpose for reporting incidents, in order to strengthen the argument that these reports should be protected from discovery. Incidents are reported to notify appropriate hospital personnel and the professional liability carrier(s) of potential claims. The incident report is the first step to claims investigation and should contain information that becomes part of a claims file. A second reason for reporting incidents is to allow remedial action to be put into effect that will prevent similar incidents from occurring in the future, thereby meeting loss prevention and quality assurance goals.

CONFIDENTIALITY

In determining whether hospital incident reports are discoverable, courts have taken several factors into consideration.

Attorney-Client Privilege

One factor courts consider when the release of information is in question is whether or not there is an attorney-client privilege. Confidential communications from a client to an attorney for the purpose of seeking legal assistance are protected from discovery by the attorney-client privilege. Courts have extended this privilege to protect communications between the attorney and a member of a "control group" authorized to make decisions for the corporation with respect to legal matters about which the attorney was consulted. In a unanimous opinion, using the Federal Rules of Evidence, the United States Supreme Court expanded the traditional attorney-client privilege to include communications between nonmanagement personnel and the corporate attorney, when the employees were acting within the scope of their employment.[1]

As well, state courts have generally recognized the traditional scope of the attorney-client privilege to include communications between a corporate employee and the corporate attorney when the "communication relates to a fact (about) which the attorney was informed by his client . . . for the purpose of securing primarily either an opinion of law, legal services, or assistance in some legal proceeding."[2] For example, the California Supreme Court held that

> where the employee's connection with the matter grows out of his employment to the extent that his report or statement is required in the ordinary course of the corporation's business, the employee is no longer an independent witness, and his statement or report is that of the employer; if the employer requires (by standing rule or otherwise) that the employee make a report, the privilege of that report is to be determined by the employer's purpose in requiring the same; . . . if the employer directs the making of the report for confidential transmittal by its attorney, the communication may be privileged.[3]

Communications, including hospital incident reports, made by hospital staff to the hospital's professional liability insurer are protected in most jurisdictions under the attorney-client privilege.[4]

In one example of a case in which the incident report was not protected by the attorney-client privilege, the report had been labeled "Patient incident report—not a notice of loss—for loss prevention purposes only." Reports were being sent on a monthly basis to the insurance carrier, rather than being sent immediately after incidents. In a second case in which an incident report was not protected, copies of reports were sent to the hospital administrator and the director of nurses, and a third copy was attached to the patient's chart.[5]

These cases suggest that when the primary purpose of the incident report is to provide information to the hospital's attorney or the liability insurer responsible for defending the hospital or its employee in a malpractice claim, the attorney-client privilege should protect the reports from discovery. Evidence of the purpose of the report may be seen in whether employees are told that the reports are made in confidence, and in how the hospital treats the report once it is received. If reports are used primarily for data collection, are placed in a patient's medical record, or are not treated confidentially, they will probably not be protected from discovery by the attorney-client privilege, even if a copy of the report is sent to the insurer or attorney.[6]

Attorney Work Product

A second doctrine under which incident reports have been found to be protected from discovery is the attorney work product privilege. In jurisdictions that have adopted the Federal Rules of Civil Procedure, the attorney work product doctrine is codified in Rule 26(b)(3), which was drafted from guidelines set forth by the United States Supreme Court in *Hickman v. Taylor*.[7]

In determining whether hospital incident reports are protected by the attorney work product doctrine, courts look at why the reports were prepared. Reports must be prepared in anticipation of litigation if the attorney work product privilege is to protect them from discovery.[8]

The work product doctrine only offers qualified immunity from discovery. If the plaintiff is able to show a substantial need for obtaining the information and that undue hardship would ensue in obtaining the documents' equivalents, the documents, even if attorney work product, may be discoverable. An effective response by defendant hospitals to this argument by plaintiffs is that the individuals who completed the incident reports are available for deposition and testimony at trial.[9]

The risk manager should have an agreement with the professional liability insurer(s) that in-house investigation will be conducted on certain categories of incidents. That agreement should be confirmed in writing.

Hospital personnel should be instructed to verbally report serious incidents to the hospital attorney or risk manager immediately after the patient's needs have been addressed. To facilitate this reporting, an on-call list of risk management or hospital attorney staff should be distributed to necessary individuals so that serious incidents occurring during off-hours may be reported promptly and hospital personnel can receive the advice and guidance they need in order to appropriately respond to the incident.

More "routine" incidents, such as medication errors, falls, and the like, that are completed on hospital incident report forms should be received by risk management within 24 hours of the incident's occurrence.

Hospital personnel should be instructed, and risk management forms should be designed, to communicate the facts about the incident, not the opinions or conclusions of the person writing the report.

All incidents should be entered into a database for loss prevention and quality assurance programs.

All reports should be sent, as soon as possible, to the professional liability insurance carrier as notice of claims or potential claims.

Incidents that identify a clear liability situation, as well as incidents in which patients have been seriously injured, should be handled along the following lines:

Initially:

1. Open a case file.
2. Record personal data about the patient: name, age, address, family members, occupation, and medical insurance status.
3. Document the patient's current medical condition, reason for being in the hospital (admission, clinic visit), and underlying medical condition
4. Read (copy if possible) pertinent portions of the patient's medical record.
5. List the names of individuals involved in the incident, their job titles, and how they can be reached (telephone number, department).
6. Safeguard equipment, products, or other evidence involved in the incident.
7. Notify the billing department(s) to hold bills temporarily.
8. Have a discussion with the patient's primary physician about what occurred during the incident, the prognosis for the patient, the patient's and/or family's attitude about what happened, what the physician thinks would be appropriate with respect to billing the patient,

who should contact the patient and/or family, and whether or not the patient is entitled to any other compensation because of the incident. (This includes a quick assessment of whether or not the physician, nurse, or other hospital employee was negligent and may be liable for the patient's injury.)

It is important for the patient and/or family to be told about the incident, if an injury occurred, as soon and as accurately as possible. It is best if this is done by the patient's primary physician. In talking with the patient and/or the patient's family, the physician should be reminded to not be overly reassuring about the patient's outcome, nor to speculate about what occurred and why it occurred. It may also be wise, when serious incidents occur, for the entire treatment team—nurses, physicians, and other patient care staff—to meet to discuss and clarify who the primary contact person will be to respond to the patient's and/or family's questions concerning the incident. It is important that the patient and/or family not hear misinformation or contradicting information.

The information obtained in the investigation should be communicated as soon as possible to the professional liability insurance carrier, and a joint decision should be made about how to proceed with the management of the situation. The decision about how to proceed should be communicated to the patient's primary physician. If a nurse or other hospital employee is primarily involved in the incident, that employee should also be informed about how the situation is being managed.

Once the patient is represented by an attorney, the hospital and its health care providers involved in the incident should refer all questions and leave all interactions to the professional liability carrier or the attorney the carrier retains to represent them. In-house evaluation of the claim by experts in the area is important in evaluating how defensible the case would be in court. Such an evaluation should be offered to the defense attorney and should be coordinated by the hospital risk management or attorney's staff.

If a product or piece of equipment is involved, it should be tested by an outside facility. The basic facts (not including any identifying patient information) of incidents involving equipment or products should be reported to the United States Pharmacopeia, 12601 Twinbrook Parkway, Rockville, Maryland 20852, as well as to the manufacturer of the product or equipment.

Loss Prevention/Quality Assurance

Data from all incidents should be entered into a database for analysis and presentation to the risk management and/or quality assurance committee(s) to determine if changes in policies, procedures, in-service education, or other areas are necessary as remedial measures.

Claim Control

Any communications with the patient and/or family, as well as any billing adjustments, must have the approval of the professional liability insurance carrier prior to being done. Discussions with the patient and/or the patient's family should be kind and straightforward. If appropriate, bills should be adjusted.

The patient and/or family should know whom to contact if they have further questions, concerns, or demands.

The hospital attorney, risk management staff member, or claims adjuster should make clear to the patient and/or family what will be done (if anything) to compensate the patient for the injury that occurred and what will be expected from the patient or family in return, such as signing a release and settlement agreement in return for writing off bills.

If the incident results in a lawsuit, the member of the risk management or hospital attorney's staff who initially investigated and managed the claim should continue to be the liaison with the defense attorney and hospital personnel involved in the claim. This arrangement will foster a closer, more confident working relationship between hospital personnel and the risk management or hospital attorney's office, which will lead to better reporting, better loss prevention, and better investigation and management of future claims.

NOTES

1. Charles David Creech, "Comment, The Medical Review Committee Privilege: A Jurisdictional Survey," *North Carolina Law Review* 67 no. 1 (Nov. 1988): 216.

2. Ibid., p. 217.

3. Ibid.

4. Ibid., p. 218.

5. Ibid., pp. 220–21.

6. Ibid., p. 222.

7. Ibid., p. 223.

8. Ibid., pp. 223–24.

9. Ibid., p. 224.

10. Ibid., p. 219.

11. Ibid., p. 222.

12. Ibid.

13. But see *Hospital Law Manual,* "Medical Records," 4–5 Hospital Incident Reports, March 1988-Update, p. g. reporting *Sims v. Knollwood Park Hospital,* 511 So. 2d 154 (Ala. 1987) in which the Alabama Supreme Court allowed discovery of a hospital incident report that had been submitted to the hospital's legal office. The court held that the report was documentation of the witness's impressions and observations, not those of the attorney, and would not protect it from discovery as attorney work product or under the attorney-client privilege.

14. Hospital Law Manual, "Medical Records," 4–5 Hospital Incident Reports, Rockville. Md.: Aspen Publishers, Inc., 1986, p. 78.

chapter 16

Investigation Strategies for Early Resolution

Pamela Ann Lockowitz

Conflict is defined as a disagreement or an emotional tension resulting from an incompatible inner need or drive. In the health care setting, conflict may arise when client expectations are not met by the professionals entrusted with a patient's health and well-being. It is not uncommon for health care professionals to avoid conflict after an untoward occurrence, particularly when human tragedy and suffering are at the center of the dispute. Not knowing what to say to an injured patient or grieving family is an unfortunate reality that tends to fuel these situations. After an untoward event, if clients' questions and concerns are not satisfactorily answered, they frequently believe that their only means of redress is through the existing legal system. Unfortunately, this system is usually costly for both hospital and client and is often unduly cumbersome. It is also fraught with uncertainties and delays for all involved parties. Developing alternative means for dealing with conflict is in clients' and health care provider's best interest. The risk manager must be a key player in the early resolution of these conflicts and should act as the catalyst.

This chapter will examine methods available to health care risk managers that may be appropriately referred to as alternative dispute resolution methods. Properly utilized, these methods will allow the risk manager better control over claims asserted against a facility and will improve the risk manager's ability to control the associated financial loss.

EARLY DETECTION OF POTENTIAL CLAIMS

Key to the risk manager's ability to control loss is an ability to recognize potential claims early. It is important to remember that a risk manager cannot be effective if forced to act independently of the health care professionals and staff of the institution. An effective risk manager first must develop a close working relationship with the persons who provide hands-on patient care. These professionals are often the first to realize that an untoward event has occurred. As stated in the preceding chapter, the risk manager must establish an open line of communication so that he or she is advised of events as soon as possible. The risk manager must develop an occurrence reporting system that these professionals understand and are willing to utilize. Then, education must be provided to enable staff to determine which instances warrant the completion of an administrative incident report. A good general rule of thumb is that staff should complete an occurrence report any time an unexpected outcome results from a therapeutic or diagnostic procedure. (See Exhibit 16-1.) Providing staff with a list of reportable injuries is often helpful. (This information is discussed in greater detail in those chapters dealing with occurrence screening and in those addressing department-specific reportable incidents.)

EVALUATING LIABILITY AND COSTS

Upon receipt of the occurrence report, the risk manager must evaluate and respond to the situation. First, identification of the potential or actual liability associated with the incident at hand is necessary to determine if a

---

Exhibit 16-1 Staff Notification of Reportable Incidents

MEMORANDUM

TO: All Professional Staff
FROM: Risk Manager

An administrative occurrence report must be completed any time a patient suffers an unexpected outcome while under our care and treatment. Reports are required for but should not be limited to the following injuries:

1. unexplained or unexpected death
2. brain damage
3. spinal cord injury
4. nerve injury or neurologic deficit
5. loss of limb, sensory organ, or reproductive organ
6. disfigurement
7. unexpected return to surgery

Please complete a report and forward it to the office of Risk Management as soon as possible after the untoward event.

potential problem indeed exists. To do this, the risk manager must understand what the prevailing standard of care is and must determine whether the standard was met. It is likely that the best source of information to assist in determining this standard will be the in-house clinical management team (or individual, department-specific quality review committees). This team may include head nurses, nursing supervisors, division chairs, and department managers. These professionals should be able to assist the risk manager with the early investigation and evaluation of untoward occurrences. They should gather factual information from hands-on caregivers and define for the risk manager the applicable standard of care. They should also be able to comment on whether they believe a breach in standard care was the likely cause of the patient's injury. These causation issues are an important element of the risk manager's loss analysis. Since this investigation analysis process will yield very sensitive, confidential information, it would be prudent for the risk manager to ask local defense counsel how to protect this information from discovery if the case cannot be resolved in the early stages and goes on to court.

If the risk manager determines that the case has merit and that early resolution would be advisable, he or she must then attempt to place a value on the case. Certain categories of damages require specific evaluation. Special damages represent an actual out-of-pocket loss to the claimant. These may include, but are not limited to, hospital costs, lost earnings, nursing home care, and medications. It is important to remember that past, present, and future damages are part of this evaluation. These estimates are generally straightforward. On the other hand, the general damages associated with a given case are much more difficult to calculate. General damages should include remuneration for emotional injury, pain, mental anguish, and other similarly related complaints.

DEVELOPING THE CLAIM MANAGEMENT STRATEGY

Once the risk manager has evaluated the liability aspects of the case, calculated the associated damages, and placed a dollar value on the injury, he or she is ready to develop a claim management strategy. At this point a number of options for early resolution are available. One is to do nothing: If the risk manager believes that the incident caused no serious harm or injury and further believes that the incident will be forgotten, he or she may elect to continue to watch but not to approach the patient or the family at that time. A second option is to arrange a meeting with the patient or the patient's family to discuss the conflict and how best the patient or family believes it can be resolved. The risk manager may wish to make this contact alone or may request that one of the clinical managers participate in the meeting. Based on the findings of the meeting, it may then be necessary to bring in additional persons (e.g., structured settlement specialist, rehabilitation counselor, equipment specialist), who can assist with early resolution.

The approach to each case obviously must be individualized, and the players may vary accordingly. The important thing to remember is that the approach to the client should be consistent, open, and honest. There is nothing more frustrating to an injured patient (or one who perceives himself or herself to be injured) than to receive multiple and/or different explanations from a variety of different hospital representatives.

During the conversation with the client, the risk manager should solicit information concerning the patient's perception of the injury, the cause of the injury, and the type of retribution being sought. When the risk manager gains some insight into the feelings of the patient or the family, he or she will be in a better position to elect the appropriate claim management strategy. This is important since there are a number of different conflict resolution strategies available to the risk manager.

The risk manager may wish to offer a bill write-off or an adjustment to the patient's hospital bill. Knowing that there will be no out-of-pocket expenses associated with the incident is sometimes all that the patient or family desires. However, before this approach is offered, the risk manager should understand how such a resolution is viewed in the local jurisdiction and, related to that, should consult with local counsel regarding the effect of such a write-off. Depending on the amount of money involved, the risk manager may also wish to consult with counsel regarding the pros and cons of obtaining a release. In certain instances, the requirement that a patient sign a release may raise unnecessary concern on the part of the patient, but in others it may be absolutely necessary in order to protect the interests of the hospital.

Another approach to conflict resolution is to offer the patient the needed services required for returning the patient to a preinjury status, free of charge. For example, if a fall from bed results in a broken arm and three months of physical therapy, it may be prudent to provide the therapy at no charge. Again, depending upon the amount of money associated with this transaction, the risk manager may want to obtain a release. In general, and when possible, it is best to obtain a signed release. The risk manager, however, must weigh the possible negative effect that a release form may have on early negotiations.

If neither of these alternatives is viable, the risk manager may want to negotiate a monetary settlement with the patient or the family, prior to the involvement of an attorney. In this instance, the risk manager must gain the patient's confidence and persuade him or her that hiring an attorney will not necessarily lead to a better settlement. In fact, less may actually be recovered because of the costs associated with legal fees. It is also important to emphasize that the legal process can be protracted and the patient may not see any financial recovery for years following the incident.

With a monetary settlement, there are a number of different approaches the risk manager can utilize. A cash settlement is an option but is not always in the best interest of the claimant. Although the settlement is not taxable, any proceeds from invested funds are taxable at the claimant's current tax rate. Furthermore, studies have shown that the proceeds from cash settlements are expended within the first five years following the incident. This can be particularly detrimental for the claimant who has long-term financial needs related to an injury.

An option that should be explored if the settlement is expected to be large and if the patient expects to have long-term expenses associated with the injury is a structured settlement or annuity. Structured settlements are beneficial to both the hospital and the claimant. First, the hospital can adequately provide for the claimant's needs while spending less to resolve the loss. Second, the claimant receives the settlement, tax-free, over an extended period of time, which is consistent with how the needs for services will arise. (See Exhibit 16-2.) To implement a structured settlement, the risk manager must have established a relationship with a structured settlement firm or a specialist who has access to quality annuity marketplaces. The hospital's insurance carrier should be able to provide names of well-respected structured settlement firms.

If these attempts to resolve the loss do not prove to be successful, the risk manager might suggest to the patient that they enter into mediation or arbitration. Mediation is a process whereby the parties in conflict select a disinterested third party to assist them in reaching a mutually acceptable settlement; the mediator cannot, however, force the parties to accept a binding decision. Arbitration, on the other hand, is a process whereby both parties present their cases to a neutral third party who will offer a solution based on the facts. This can be structured to be a binding or a nonbinding arbitration. If either of these approaches is to be utilized, the risk manager should be familiar with the existing laws in his or her jurisdiction addressing mediation and arbitration proceedings.

WHEN CONFLICT MANAGEMENT HAS FAILED

If none of these attempts to resolve the conflict proves successful, the risk manager should keep an open mind and door to the claimant, for he or she may simply need some time to think about the options that have

Exhibit 16-2 Sample Settlement Proposal

	Benefit	Yield	Cost
Settlement Proposal John Jones (Age 48) Natural Life Expectancy 72 years			
Cash $25,000	$ 25,000	$ 25,000	$ 25,000
Monthly Pay $500/month for life 20-year guarantee to begin 9/1/88	120,000	144,000	55,881
Lump Sums 9/1/90 $ 5,000 9/1/95 10,000 9/1/2000 15,000 9/1/2005 20,000	50,000	50,000	24,421
	$195,000	$219,000 (Assignment Fee)	$105,302 + 500 $105,802

been offered. Given sufficient time, the claimant may decide to accept the proposal or to make a counter offer. All counter offers should be considered, and the claimant should receive a response to each of the offers as an indication that the risk manager and the institution are still very interested in early resolution of a claim. Keeping communication lines open and congenial is the first rule of successful negotiation.

Finally, be prepared for the claimant to seek the advice of counsel. The risk manager may even receive a telephone call from the claimant's attorney. In this case, the risk manager should listen to the attorney but not be put off by the call. The risk manager should also not call off all further attempts to reach a settlement with the patient simply because there is an additional player on the other side. In fact, the risk manager should continue with open dialogue to attempt to resolve the loss amicably. If, at this point, the case is successfully negotiated, a release is now imperative. If settlement is not possible, the risk manager may have to allow the case to go forward in the traditional sense, remembering that at any point along the discovery/trial continuum, a case may be ripe for settlement. Once it is evident that the case is to be litigated, it should be referred to defense counsel so that counsel can begin to work with the risk manager toward a successful resolution.

chapter 17

Understanding and Managing the Litigation Phase

Barbara J. Youngberg

There is no doubt that a successful claims management program is dependent not only on the work and skill of the hospital risk management staff (and in-house counsel) but also, to an equal and at times to a greater extent, on the quality of outside defense counsel hired to handle a case as it progresses toward final disposition (be this negotiation and settlement or trial). The importance of a good working relationship between hospital staff and defense counsel cannot be underestimated. The effectiveness of this relationship can best be maintained by having specific guidelines that all parties are aware of and that provide continual and ongoing analysis of the quality of work provided. Both parties must realize that there are specific strengths that each brings to the table in preparing a complex medical case for disposition. These strengths include

- the hospital staff's ability to evaluate the complex medical data that comprise the allegations in the case
- the professional staff of physicians and nurses, who can evaluate the alleged injury and assist the attorney in establishing (or disputing) "proximate cause" arguments
- the pre-existing relationships physicians and nurses have with colleagues who might be willing to defend the care rendered by serving as experts in the case
- defense counsel's skill in recognizing the legal impact certain allegations or situations may have on a jury or judge, which might affect the decision to settle or try a case
- defense counsel's sensitivity to jurisdictional precedent that may affect the final outcome of a case

221

- defense counsel's skill in negotiating with opposing counsel and in posturing a case for final disposition
- defense counsel's skill in trial preparation and litigation

CHOOSING DEFENSE COUNSEL

Critical to building a strong team to represent the interest of the hospital is the hiring of superior defense counsel. It is not enough to hire a defense firm that is merely "competent," as plaintiffs who feel they have been wronged or persons with devastating injuries generally hire the most superior plaintiff's counsel they can find. When a hospital faces a claim for catastrophic injury with a multimillion dollar verdict potential, it must be convinced that its representation will be as skilled as that provided to the plaintiff. Cutting costs by hiring a mediocre law firm is likely to result in severe financial losses for the hospital faced with anything but the most insignificant of lawsuits. Suggested guidelines for choosing competent counsel follow.

Remember, the most expensive, largest, or most prestigious law firm is not necessarily the best. It is important to evaluate the members of the firm who will be handling your business and not those whose names are most frequently associated with the firm.

Although many persons hiring attorneys place great importance on the education of the attorneys working in the firm (for example, hiring a firm that hires only Ivy League graduates), one must carefully evaluate the experience and success of individual members of the firm. (Obviously, a graduate from a prestigious law school who has no proven negotiation skills and who lacks trial presence will be ineffective in the handling of hospital malpractice cases.)

Ask to see not only résumés but also a list of clients, successful defense verdicts, lists of the types of cases handled by the attorneys (has the firm handled cases where brain damage to infants is alleged, or where similar catastrophic and complex injuries are verified?), and a list of the number of cases tried to verdict as compared to those settled.

Ask if any members of the firm (professional or paraprofessional) have any medical, nursing, or hospital training. It is very helpful and can be cost-effective to hire a firm that employs nurse-attorneys, physician-attorneys, and/or nurse paralegals who can expeditiously and accurately evaluate the medical issues in a case and assist in the education of other attorneys who may be called up to litigate the case.

Ask who will be responsible for the day-to-day management of a case. Well-supervised associates will be of greater value than a senior partner who is extremely skilled but too busy to pay attention to the details of the case until the day of trial. Verify that there is constant supervision of any inexperienced associates and that these attorneys are never sent out alone to handle critical aspects of the case.

Ask up front what the firm's billing procedures are. A law firm should not charge you to train their attorneys. Thus, you should determine whether the firm has a policy against "double-billing" (charging the client for work done by a junior-level associate to enable her or him to gain experience, which must be redone or done in conjunction with another higher-level associate or partner).

Show the law firm your management guidelines and verify whether they are willing to comply with them.

DEFENSE ATTORNEY CASE MANAGEMENT GUIDELINES

In most cases, outside defense counsel will be assigned a case when litigation commences or when the hospital has a strong reason to believe that it will (e.g., a letter from the plaintiff's counsel indicating an intent to litigate). There are other times when hospitals would be wise to involve defense counsel much earlier to enable them to gain control of the issues prior to the opposing counsel's doing so. This is especially true in cases where there is verified catastrophic injury or significant negative publicity associated with the facts of the case.

Assignment and Acknowledgment

An acknowledgment letter should be sent from the law firm to the representative of the hospital who will be handling the file. The letter should describe a timetable for the initial assignment of counsel to handle the case and for analysis of issues and exposure.

Designation of Counsel

Although it is quite likely that a number of attorneys in the firm will at some point participate in the preparation of a complex medical case, it is vitally important to have a designated attorney be responsible for the management of the file. That person will be the contact for hospital staff who are involved in the case and the person who directs the strategy and assigns the work related to the case.

It is not essential that the managing attorney conduct all aspects of the pretrial and discovery phases of litigation. However, the managing attorney must be aware of all significant aspects of the case as they develop, remain cognizant of major depositions, motions, and hearings, and be available (and prepared) in the event the case proceeds to trial. She or he must also be the principal negotiator in the event of settlement discussions.

The name of the attorney assigned as the managing counsel should be provided to the hospital within two weeks of acknowledgment of receipt of the case.

Initial Meeting with Hospital Representative

As soon as possible (definitely within the first month of receipt of a case), the managing attorney and any associates who plan to work on the case should meet with appropriate personnel from the hospital (risk manager and in-house counsel). Since it is important to establish a good working relationship with all parties to the lawsuit, this meeting should be aimed at introducing staff, providing an initial analysis of exposure, analyzing strengths and weaknesses, and identifying key persons who will assist the attorney in understanding the medical facts at issue. All of these facts will assist in the formulation of an initial strategy.

Defense counsel should also recognize that the hospital will be able to provide them with a wealth of expertise to assist them in understanding the facts at issue. If hospital personnel are unable to effectively or realistically analyze exposure, they can be asked to recommend someone outside of the hospital who would qualify as an expert.

This initial meeting should always take place prior to the filing of an answer to the complaint.

Providing Appropriate Documents for Hospital Files

It is essential that the hospital be provided with significant documents related to the case that have bearing on the ultimate outcome of the case. When appropriate, the hospital should be asked to assist in the preparation of these documents.

Pleadings

The hospital file should always contain a copy of the answer filed on behalf of the named defendant(s). In cases where there is significant injury or where excessive damages are alleged, the hospital may elect whether or not to receive summaries of interrogatories, depositions, any cross-claims and counterclaims, or any dispositive motions.

Damage Information

In all cases, the hospital file should contain a list of damages alleged by the plaintiff. All damages alleged should be verified by defense counsel. In controverted cases, defense counsel should provide the hospital with their analysis of exposure and, when appropriate, with possible verdict ranges for the case if it proceeds to trial. It is also helpful if defense counsel provide the hospital with a predicted settlement value for the case.

Coupled with the damage information, defense counsel should also provide, early on, an estimate of fees (including attorney fees, administrative costs, and expert witness fees). This will enable the hospital to appropriately reserve funds to pay for losses. It will also assist in making the decision of whether a case should be tried or settled.

Statutory Offers

No statutory offers are to be filed without the authorization of the hospital and/or named defendants (if they include hospital staff). If an offer is agreed upon and made, a copy of it should be forwarded to the hospital for its file.

Law and Motions

In some situations, seeking procedural remedies can have a positive effect, including termination of the action against the hospital or its employees. In considering demurrers, pretrial motions, or other procedural defenses, the hospital will rely on outside counsel's legal experience and expertise as to the chances of success and validity. If the motion to be filed deals with a material issue in the lawsuit, it should be discussed with the representative(s) from the hospital who is handling the case. If possible, any possible deleterious effects of filing the motion should also be addressed. A copy of the motion should be provided to the hospital for its file.

Cross-Claims or Third Party Actions

After complete analysis of the facts in a lawsuit, defense counsel may suggest that a cross-claim be filed. It should be recognized that in all cases where a cross-claim would be filed against a hospital physician or employee, defense counsel must consult with the hospital. Obviously, since the filing of a cross-claim against such a party could greatly complicate the defense of a case and could cause extreme political friction within the hospital, careful consideration must be given to the merits of filing such an action. Defense counsel must recognize that even though filing such a complaint may be legally sound, it may not be in the best interest of the hospital to pursue such an action. Defense counsel should prepare arguments to assist the hospital in making this difficult decision. If a decision is made to proceed with such an action, a copy of the pleadings should be sent to the hospital prior to their filing.

Depositions

The hospital will rely upon the experience of defense counsel as to the timing of the taking of all depositions. If a hospital staff member or physician is being deposed, defense counsel should notify the hospital representative (risk manager or in-house counsel) well in advance so that his or her attendance at the deposition may be assured. Defense counsel must also be willing to spend time with the hospital employee or physician prior to the deposition to give him or her the opportunity to review the records, ask questions, and in general prepare for this experience. If the law firm routinely summarizes all depositions, copies of the summaries should be sent to the hospital. The deposition of the principal causation expert should be sent to the hospital in its entirety to enable its complete review by clinical in-house experts. It is not necessary to send the hospital copies of depositions that have no material bearing on the facts at issue.

In cases where ex-employees are being subpoenaed for depositions, the risk manager should take responsibility for locating these persons and should review their personnel files. This will assist in recognizing potential hostile witnesses and may minimize the cost of finding the witnesses, as often the hospital has knowledge of the persons' whereabouts.

Initial Investigation and Discovery

Too often, defense counsel forgets the value of the input of the hospital in this phase of the legal process. The hospital will provide defense counsel with a complete copy of the medical record of the patient and, when appropriate, will advise counsel of the existence of other records that may be relevant to the plaintiff's case. The hospital will review the record and ask that the managing attorney also review the record—in its entirety—so that a meeting can be held early in the discovery process to clarify terms and issues and to establish the appropriate standard of care. At this time the hospital will also share with defense counsel any potential hidden problems (such as disciplinary action taken against an employee, peer review problems with the physician, etc.), which may affect the way the case is postured.

Continued Case Development

Throughout the course of trial preparation, defense counsel should remain in contact with the hospital representative working on the file. If at any time new facts become known to counsel that materially alter the strategy agreed upon, it will be incumbent upon the managing attorney to immediately notify the hospital. Any offers to settle should also be conveyed to the hospital as soon as made.

TIMETABLE FOR REPORTING

The hospital realizes that in many jurisdictions there is an extreme backlog in the courts, making it very difficult to move a case expeditiously to trial. Nevertheless, we feel that attorneys must remain cognizant of the importance of reporting the ongoing preparation of a case, which will enable a hospital to determine whether a case should be tried or settled. (See Exhibit 17-1.) In cases where liability is clear and injury is verified, it may well be in the best interest of the hospital to effect an early settlement, thus minimizing defense costs and staff anxiety. Sufficient discovery can be completed early on, enabling defense counsel and the hospital to formulate an opinion as to the probable disposition and value of a lawsuit.

EXPECTATIONS OF OUTSIDE DEFENSE COUNSEL

Preliminary Meeting and Report

As soon as an assignment is received, counsel should attempt to meet with appropriate persons from the hospital to formulate a response to the

Exhibit 17-1 Reporting Timetable

Within 2 Weeks
- acknowledgment of assignment
- meeting arranged with hospital staff
- preparation and filing of an answer (copy provided to hospital)

Within 30 Days
- designation of managing attorney
- initial analysis of exposure following meeting with hospital staff and named defendants
- identification of litigants and their relationship to the incident
- outline of initial strategy

Within 60 Days
- contact established with plaintiff attorney to discuss case
- identification of potential experts to support defense position (this identification is provided to the hospital only)
- analysis of relevant state statutes and loss trends that might affect evaluation
- identification of possible third party defendants, along with an analysis of their exposure
- analysis of applicable collateral source payments
- assessment of capabilities of opposing counsel
- outline of future discovery

Within 90 Days
- analysis of interrogatories and discovery completed to date
- analysis of liability, settlement, and verdict range
- extent of contribution expected from codefendants
- statements of damages and how they will be verified
- outline of continued discovery

All future reports should follow at regular intervals and should address all material issues as they relate to the development of the case and the posturing of it for trial or settlement.

pleadings and to formulate a basic outline defining the direction of discovery. Following this meeting, the hospital should be provided with a copy of counsel's response to the pleadings and a written report delineating counsel's overall sense of the direction of the case.

Six-Month Evaluation

Within a six-month period a reasonably sound evaluation can be completed, which will assist the hospital in appropriately reserving a case and in preparing for the direction it will likely take (dismissal vs. settlement vs. trial). At the end of the sixth month, the hospital should be provided with a report that discusses information related to verification of injury, the plaintiff's damages, proof of allegations, vulnerabilities, the potential liability of the insured, potential third party defendants, and plans for future activity. It is also very helpful at this point for defense counsel to comment on the skill, experience, and expertise of the plaintiff's attorney handling this case. (This is especially true if plaintiff's counsel is known to be extremely aggressive and successful in the area of medical malpractice.) At this stage of preparation, defense counsel should also have a plan for completing discovery, which includes a timing of activities. Significant delays in this process should also be explained.

Supplemental Reports

The hospital expects to be kept informed of any new developments in a case as they occur. It is not necessary that defense counsel send monthly status reports indicating no activity, but it is critical that the hospital remain current on the developments of each case. The hospital may wish to determine on a case-by-case basis which files it would like monthly or bimonthly reports on (e.g., cases that pose a substantial financial threat to the hospital may require monthly status reports).

VOLUNTARY AND MANDATORY SETTLEMENT CONFERENCE REQUIREMENTS

It is essential that the hospital be aware of all voluntary and mandatory settlement conference scheduled to take place, well in advance of the dates scheduled. Prior to a conference's being held, defense counsel will meet with hospital personnel to discuss relevant issues as they relate to settlement. These might include the decision to settle, the use of a structured settlement or annuity for settlement, the advantages of early settlement, the likely verdict range, and the likely settlement figure. At this preconference meeting, the hospital will advise counsel as to what, if any, portion of the settlement will be paid by insurance, as opposed to what will be borne by the hospital.

During the preconference meeting with the hospital, defense counsel should be prepared to discuss the merits and weaknesses of the case and to recommend the position the hospital should take. It would be most helpful if counsel provided a list of similar cases in the jurisdiction that had been resolved either through trial or settlement, so that the hospital can make a decision as to the wisdom of early settlement.

Defense counsel should insist that the plaintiff and/or his or her representative be present at any and all discussions related to settlement. (Often the plaintiff finds it very difficult to turn down even a minimal amount of money when faced with the fact that at trial they may receive nothing.)

EXPERT WITNESSES AND EXPERT REVIEWERS

Again, it should be emphasized that the hospital wishes to be integrally involved in the procurement and use of experts in all of its cases. Though counsel is often in a better position to identify experts who are reputed to be dishonest or hired guns, the hospital is often in the best position to identify persons who might have particular expertise in a subspecialty, which could be the pivotal issue in a case. The hospital is often also in a position to identify offensive or negative personality characteristics of experts, which might taint or color the testimony rendered. Identifying the best expert is often the key to a successful defense.

A verbal report should be solicited from the expert prior to a written report, and a final copy of the written report should be sent to the hospital to become part of the hospital file.

In all cases, the hospital should be advised when depositions of the plaintiff's expert witnesses are being taken. It is often very effective to have a defendant physician, nurse, or hospital representative present to remind this expert whom she or he is testifying against.

TRIAL PROCEDURE

Defense counsel must notify the hospital of all impending trial dates so that a representative of the hospital can be present throughout the trial. Prior to the trial, defense counsel should also prepare a complete analysis of the issues remaining for trial, the substance of the testimony of the experts, the skill of the experts testifying, the emotional underpinnings of the trial, and the likelihood of prevailing at trial. A list of all witnesses who are likely to be called should also be provided to enable the hospital to arrange with its departments for staff time off.

Defense counsel should arrange for witnesses to be briefed on appropriate trial demeanor and protocol. They should give witnesses the opportunity to review their depositions and explain to them the testimony that is likely to be offered against them. They should be cautioned against feeling compelled to answer all questions, especially if they have limited knowledge or are unaware of the correct answer.

POST-TRIAL MOTIONS

The hospital should be advised of any and all post-trial motions filed against or on behalf of the defendants. Prior to the filing of motions, the managing attorney should meet with the hospital representative and the named defendants and discuss the rationale and implications for the filing of the motions. A copy of the motion should be given to the hospital at the time it is filed.

chapter 18

Summation: What Can Be Learned from the Process?

Barbara J. Youngberg

The settlement of a large lawsuit or the conclusion of a long trial can often bring either a sense of great relief or incredible despair for hospital staff. Despite the outcome, if a case has consumed a great deal of staff time and has caused a great deal of agony, parties may feel the need to quickly forget what has taken place prior to the final resolution. Despite the desire to put the past behind, it is important to recognize the benefits of careful analysis of the process that lead to the outcome. What is gained from this analysis can then be used to prepare for future settlements and lawsuits. The information gained from this process can also be used to drive quality assurance and risk management efforts and to provide topics for staff education programs.

PARTICIPANTS IN EVALUATION

Who should participate in this evaluation will be determined by the nature of the lawsuit, the parties involved, the magnitude of the outcome, and the resultant effects the resolution of the case may have on staff members. Risk management and administrative staff should determine the appropriateness of involving various persons in the process. The following list should assist in that determination:

1. all named parties in the lawsuit and hospital staff who were called to testify or who were deposed prior to settlement
2. in-house risk management and legal staff (generally the most appropriate people to act as group facilitators since they often are the people most familiar with all of the elements of the case)

3. a senior administrative representative (since a large settlement or verdict often has many financial implications for a hospital and also, especially, if disciplinary action is to be taken following the process)
4. the director of marketing (since sensational cases or those generating a great deal of publicity can do a great deal of harm, and damage the reputation of even the finest hospital)
5. the attorney who handled the case or a senior partner from the defense firm involved in the case (especially—and probably best only—when the performance of defense counsel is evaluated)
6. any other hospital personnel who were involved in the process or whom the results might affect

TOPICS FOR DISCUSSION

The session may begin by allowing participants in the litigation to describe feelings, frustrations, and questions that may have arisen as the result of the litigation. Once these items have been discussed, the facilitator should focus on the significant aspects of the case. A checklist can be used by the facilitator to review the various elements of the case (Exhibit 18-1), but at the very least, the discussion should focus on the following elements:

- Did review of the issues surrounding the case lead to the conclusion that there was evidence of negligence? If so, what was done from a quality standpoint to ensure that a similar act of negligence would not be repeated? Also, if the presence of negligence and the verification of injury were confirmed, what, if anything, could have been done to more expeditiously resolve the litigation? Were reasonable attempts made to settle, prior to spending significant money on legal fees for a case where the value of settlement was known early on?

- Was jurisdictional precedent evaluated prior to setting a strategy for resolution? Could the final outcome have been predicted, based on similar cases within the jurisdiction?

- Were all opportunities to bring third parties' claims explored (equipment companies, drug companies, outside consultants, etc.), and were parties, if appropriate, added to the litigation?

- Were the emotional underpinnings of the case evaluated properly, and were these factors considered prior to developing a strategy? Did the emotional elements appear to sway the jury in its final decision?

- If negligence was not identified by hospital staff, was the case appropriately reviewed by an outside expert who might offer a nonbiased

Exhibit 18-1 Checklist for Post Resolution Evaluation Process

1. Name of case _____

2. Brief summary of facts _____

3. Hospital employees involved _____

4. Physicians involved _____

5. Act(s) of negligence alleged _____

6. Injury alleged _____

7. Was injury verified? _____
8. Was proximate cause determination made? _____
9. Defense experts in the case _____

10. Defense attorney for the case _____

11. Plaintiff experts in the case _____

12. Plaintiff attorney for the case _____

13. Outcome of the case _____

14. Damages paid, if any _____

15. Case settled via:
    [ ] cash payment   [ ] forgiveness of bill
    [ ] structured settlement/annuity   [ ] other
16. QA/RM information gained from this case:
    Hospital unit or department _____
    Policies/procedures involved _____

    Corrective action taken _____

    Disciplinary action taken _____

17. Evaluation of defense counsel _____

18. Additional comments:

impression of the care rendered? Was that person's opinion given consideration, if it differed from the original impressions?

- When experts have been used in a case, it is important to evaluate the credentials and performance of each. Was the expert the best-qualified person available? Did the expert hold up well during direct and cross-examination? Was the plaintiff's expert able to discredit the defense expert? (Exhibit 18-2 shows a form that can be used to create a permanent file on all experts who were part of a hospital trial. This will become a valuable resource when attempting to locate an expert for defense of future hospital cases or to check on the prior testimony, credentials, and expertise of the plaintiff's experts.)
- Was a senior partner involved in all phases of the trial and settlement? If an associate was involved, was supervision apparent? Was defense counsel consistently prepared for every deposition and for all phases of the trial? Was counsel effective to the jury or judge, and did he or she evidence competence equal to or greater than opposing counsel?
- Were the damages in the case appropriately evaluated? Was the hospital's case prepared with the assistance of a damage expert (economist, rehabilitation specialist, structured settlement specialist)?
- Were the witnesses and hospital staff appropriately prepared for the process? Were they familiar with hospital policies and procedures, and did the staff support the operation of the hospital?
- Were the hospital policies in place at the time of the incident appropriate? Could a different policy or procedure have prevented the injury? Were any policies changed, or were new policies created, as a result of the incident? Has their effectiveness been evaluated?

ANALYZING THE END RESULT OF A CASE

After this evaluation has been performed, participants in the evaluation can then attempt to determine why the results occurred. Often this is a very simple process; for example, if liability is easy to establish and if the injury is verified, it will not be surprising to anyone that a verdict or settlement is reached on behalf of the plaintiff. If, however, those elements are not present, the evaluation will have to analyze all of the factual elements of the case to reach a conclusion as to why the case resolved as it did, which can be very enlightening for hospital staff. Some of the elements to be considered in drawing this conclusion (and that can also be used to

Exhibit 18-2 Expert Witness Analysis Form

---

1. Name of expert _____
2. Expert's specialty _____
3. Expert's advanced degree _____
4. Additional credentials _____
   _____
   _____
   _____

5. Expert's place of employment _____
   _____

6. Name of case in which involved _____
   _____

7. Was expert testifying on behalf of the
   [ ] plaintiff
   [ ] defendant
8. Is copy of deposition or testimony on file?
   [ ] yes
   [ ] no
9. How would you rate the testimony/demeanor of the expert at trial and during depositions?
   [ ] excellent
   [ ] good
   [ ] fair
   [ ] poor
10. Was the testimony rendered consistent with the expert's expertise?
    [ ] yes
    [ ] no
11. Did the expert cite any articles or books written by him or her that directly supported the testimony rendered?
    [ ] yes
    [ ] no
12. Has the expert testified for a large number of cases?
    [ ] yes
    [ ] no
    If yes, approximate number if known _____
13. Does expert testify primarily for:
    [ ] plaintiff
    [ ] defendant
    [ ] either
14. Would you consider using this person again as an expert?
    [ ] yes
    [ ] no
15. Please describe any unique aspects of the testimony rendered or of the expert's personal style that might influence your decision to use the expert again.

---

drive risk management educational programs) are covered in the following queries:

- Was sloppy, incomplete, or falsified documentation any part of this case? Could staff have done anything differently when documenting aspects of the patient's care to more positively affect the outcome?
- Were communication failures cited by any parties in the lawsuit, and were these failures directly related to the actual/perceived injury suffered by the patient?
- Were staffing shortages or incompetent staff issues raised in support of why the injury occurred?
- Was there evidence of staff divisiveness in any part of the pretrial, trial, or settlement proceedings?
- Did hospital policy and procedure contribute to the injury, or could a hospital policy or procedure—had it been in place—prevented the injury?
- Was there clear evidence to support an employee or staff physician in the hospital?

Obviously, the key to making this process of review a meaningful one is to make it thorough. Clearly, a hospital will want to put the negative aspects of a catastrophic case behind it, but it must be cautioned to do so only after having reviewed all of the aspects of the care rendered and the defense provided. After this review has been completed, the hospital must use the information learned to prevent future, similar incidents from occurring.

Glossary

Actuarial study An analysis performed by a recognized actuary that determines appropriate funding levels required for operation of a self-insurance trust.

Aggregate limit The maximum amount the insurer will pay during the policy period, irrespective of the policy's limit of liability.

Arbitration The hearing and determination of a case in controversy by a person either chosen by the parties in opposition or by a person appointed under statutory authority.

Broker A person who represents a buyer of insurance in negotiations with the underwriter and who serves as a consultant on various aspects of the buyer's insurance program.

Claim Demand made against a hospital or physician and/or staff for money damages, usually precipitated by an accident or incident arising during the course of treatment.

Collateral source rule A rule enabling the prevailing party to offset the damage award by the amount of money received from insurance carriers.

Contingency fee A fee for service, collectable only if the outcome is favorable to the payee.

Counter-claim A claim presented by the defendant in opposition to the claim of the plaintiff.

Cross-claim A claim brought by a defendant against a plaintiff in the same action or against a

	codefendant concerning matters related to the original petition. Its purpose is to discover facts that will aid the defense.
Deposition	Testimony (under oath) of a witness taken upon interrogatories reduced to writing and used to support or substantiate testimony offered at trial. Depositions are a very important phase of the discovery process.
Discovery	That period of time following the filing of a complaint during which the parties to the litigation attempt to gain information about all facts relevant to the litigation.
Dispositive motions	Motions heard prior to the outset of trial that result in a disposition of need for litigation and that bring about a resolution of the trial.
Errors and omissions coverage	A form of legal liability protection in which the policyholder receives protection from errors or mistakes made in some manner that caused a claimant either personal injury or financial loss.
Exposure	Term synonymous with risk: Chance of loss and that potential for liability that is coverage by insurance.
Facultative reinsurance	Reinsurance that is accepted item-by-item (or risk-by-risk) after close scrutiny. This differs from reinsurance accepted by treaty.
First-dollar coverage	Commercial insurance providing protection against the entire loss covered by the policy—without requiring the insured to pay a deductible.
General liability insurance	Coverage for liability arising out of the hazards of the premises and operations.
Hard market	A time when insurance coverage is in short supply and premiums increase for that coverage which is available.
Health Care Quality Improvement Act	Recently enacted legislative mandate requiring the reporting to a federal repository of all settlements and verdicts resulting from professional negligence.

Iatrogenic injury	An injury to a patient that is inadvertently induced by a health care professional or by the treatment provided.
Impaired aggregate limits	The total of reserves paid or outstanding on claims per policy year that might result in the hospital reaching its total self-insured obligation and require the insurer to pay on all claims.
Incurred but not reported losses (IBNR)	The liability for future payments on losses that have already occurred but have not yet been reported to the insurer. This definition may be extended to include expected future development on claims already reported.
Insurance pooling	A joint insurance operation in which participants assume a predetermined interest in all aspects of the program. The participants in the pool share proportionately in the premiums, losses, expenses, and profits.
Interrogatories	Written questions prepared by one party in litigation to be answered by the opposing party. The answers to these questions serve as evidence to support or refute the facts at issue in a trial.
Malpractice	Professional misconduct, improper discharge of professional duties, or failure to meet the standard of care of a professional, resulting in harm to another.
Mediation	Intervention between parties in conflict to promote reconciliation, settlement, or compromise.
Pleadings	The formal allegations by the parties involved in a lawsuit that delineate the claims and defenses of each party and that request judgment by the court prior to resolution.
Professional liability insurance	Coverage for liability arising from the rendering of or failure to render professional services.
Quality assurance	The discipline that focuses on aspects of clinical care within a hospital, in an attempt to identify human and system errors.

Risk financing

The science of evaluating all possible elements of an institution's financial exposure—utilizing prospective and retrospective data—and developing a vehicle for investment or money management that will allow for the dollars needed in the future to pay for the risk to be available. (Risk financing includes the purchase of insurance, the operation of a self-insurance trust, financial investments, etc.)

Risk management

Originally defined by the American Hospital Association as the "science for the identification, evaluation, and treatment of the risk of financial loss." Risk management now also encompasses the evaluation and monitoring of clinical practice to recognize and prevent patient injury.

Risk purchasing group

Any group that decides to buy, on a group basis, liability insurance in compliance with the Federal Risk Retention Act.

Risk Retention Act

A federal law enacted in 1981 as a response to the rising cost and, at times, the unavailability of commercial insurance that was experienced during the 1970s. In part, this Act facilitates self-insuring against losses through risk retention groups and allows for group purchasing of commercial insurance.

Soft market

A time when the insurance marketplace sees an increase in available coverage and a stabilization or decrease in premiums.

Index